Anatomy & Physiology Essentials

Fourth Edition

Peter Reuter, M.D., Ph.D.
Department of Rehabilitation Sciences
Marieb College of Health & Human Services
Florida Gulf Coast University

Valerie Weiss, M.D., M.S.
Department of Rehabilitation Sciences
Marieb College of Health & Human Services
Florida Gulf Coast University

▶ Reuter Academic Publishing ◀

...Essentials 4th ed.

Development, design, and production management: Reuter Academic Publishing

Copyright © 2020 Reuter Academic Publishing. All rights reserved.

Copyright © 2020 Peter Reuter on all illustrations provided.

Copyright © 2020 Valerie Weiss on all illustrations provided.

This publication is protected by Copyright and permission should be obtained from the publisher prior to any prohibited reproduction, storage in a retrieval system, or transmission in any form or by any means, electronic, digital, mechanical, photocopying, recording, or likewise.

To obtain permission(s) to use material from this work, please submit a written request to

>   Reuter Academic Publishing
>   12721 Dresden Court
>   Fort Myers, FL 33912
>   USA
>   Email: reutermedical@comcast.net

For more information on this and other books visits
www.reuteracademicpublishing.com

ISBN-13: 978-1-7346811-0-9

About the Authors

Peter Reuter, M.D., Ph.D.

Dr. Reuter received his medical degree and his research doctorate from Johannes Gutenberg University in Mainz/Germany. After publishing his first book in early 1989, Dr. Reuter co-founded a medical magazine for students and contributed to other publications. However, he soon focused on compiling medical, dental, and scientific dictionaries and databases for print and digital publications. In 1998, Dr. Reuter moved to Florida and founded Reuter Medical Inc., a medical and scientific reference publishing company. Overall, he has authored or contributed to more than 100 dictionaries and textbooks as well as other publications published in six languages and nineteen countries.

In 2010, Dr. Reuter set out to fulfill his life-long ambition to teach at a university and to help students achieve their dream of becoming health professionals. He loves teaching undergraduate and graduate courses and tries to inspire students to push themselves to success when courses become challenging.

Dr. Reuter is the proud father of three wonderful daughters and one absolutely adorable granddaughter. When he is not teaching, reading or writing, he enjoys yoga, cycling, chocolate, fresh crispy bread, and German beer.

Valerie Weiss, M.D., M.S.

Dr. Weiss received her B.A. in visual arts from Brown University, including a year of study at the Rhode Island School of Design. She then earned an M.D. from Brown University Medical School followed by an M.S. in Medical Illustration from the Medical College of Georgia, where she further studied Anatomy and Physiology while learning to draw the human body.

Prior to becoming a professor, Dr. Weiss had her own business as a medical illustrator, providing medical illustrations to physicians, attorneys, educators, and other professionals. Her illustrations have been published in various books. Additionally, she has lectured to public and business groups about the connection between art and anatomy.

Dr. Weiss has been teaching at the university level since 2005. She previously taught at Hodges University, culminating as the Program Chair of the Health Studies Department and Associate Professor. In 2010, she was named Hodges University's Professor of the Year. In 2012, Dr. Weiss was excited about the opportunity to teach at Florida Gulf Coast University. She enjoys getting to know her FGCU students and challenging them to reach their potential.

Dr. Weiss is happily married with two beautiful, kind children and one very handsome husband. Along with spending time with her family, she enjoys running, swimming, and yoga.

A&P Essentials 4th ed.

Preface

Just like the previous editions, this fourth edition is based on a more comprehensive book, Reuter/Weiss *Principles of Anatomy & Physiology*. Our objective was to mirror the content covered in the two parts of the bigger book while still keeping the special character of Anatomy & Physiology Essentials our students have come to love and appreciate.

All chapters in this fourth edition have been revised and we added additional illustrations to improve the content even more. *Chapter 1 Introduction into Medical Terminology* is a new addition to the book. In the past, students often struggled with understanding anatomical and medical terms used in the book and in lecture as they didn't know the meaning of the terms. We hope that including this new chapter will increase the value of the book for our students.

As always, we are aware that despite all our efforts this edition still contains errors and omissions, and we encourage readers to give critical feedback so we can improve the book in future editions.

Peter Reuter
Valerie Weiss

A&P Essentials 4th ed.

Contents

	page
Chapter 1 Introduction into Medical Terminology	1
Chapter 2 Basic Sciences Review	5
Chapter 3 Introduction into Anatomy & Physiology	13
Chapter 4 Histology	23
Chapter 5 Integumentary System	27
Chapter 6 Bones & Skeletal Tissues	31
Chapter 7 Skeleton	37
Chapter 8 Joints	53
Chapter 9 Muscle Tissue	59
Chapter 10 Muscular System	67
Chapter 11 Nervous Tissue	81
Chapter 12 Central Nervous System	87
Chapter 13 Peripheral Nervous System & Reflexes	95
Chapter 14 General & Special Senses	105
Chapter 15 Endocrine System	117
Chapter 16 Cardiac Anatomy & Physiology	125
Chapter 17 Blood Vessels & Circulation	133
Chapter 18 Blood, Hemostasis, and Blood Groups	147
Chapter 19 Lymphatic System and Immunity	155
Chapter 20 Respiratory System	171
Chapter 21 Digestive System	183
Chapter 22 Urinary System	201
Chapter 23 Fluid, Electrolyte, and Acid-Base Balance	209
Chapter 24 Reproductive System and Pregnancy	215

A&P Essentials 4th ed.

Chapter 1 Introduction into Medical Terminology

A medical term may have three parts — a prefix, the word root, and a suffix.

Word Roots

- The word root of a medical term is the foundation of a word that gives it meaning. Word roots typically describe the part of the body or organ involved. For example: **cardi** means *heart* and **gastr** means *stomach*.
- Word roots are usually combined with a vowel at the end (often an "o") so that a suffix beginning with a consonant can be added. When word roots are written in this way, they are called **combining forms**. For example: **cardi(o)** means *heart* and **gastr(o)** means *stomach*.

Table 1.1 Combining Forms

Combining Form	Meaning	Example(s)
alg(o)-, alge-, algesi(o)-	pain	*myalgia* = pain in a muscle
arthr(o)-	joint	*arthritis* = inflammation of a joint
bacteri(o)-	bacteria	*bacteriuria* = bacteria in the urine
cerebr(o)-	cerebrum	*cerebrovascular* = relating to the blood vessels of the brain
cyan(o)-	blue	*cyanosis* = blue discoloration of the skin from a lack of oxygen
dermat(o)-, derm(o)-	skin	*dermatologist* = physician who specializes in diagnosing and treating disorders of the skin
erythr(o)-	red	*erythrocyte* = red blood cell
gluc(o)-	sugar, glucose	*glucosuria* = sugar in the urine
leuk(o)-	white	*leukemia* = a white blood cell cancer
melan(o)-	black	*melanocyte* = a cell responsible for producing skin pigment
myel(o)-	spinal cord	*myelopathy* = disease affecting the spinal cord
pancreat(o)-	pancreas	*pancreatitis* = inflammation of the pancreas
poli(o)-	gray	*poliomyelitis* = inflammation of the gray matter of the spinal cord

Prefixes

- A prefix is added to the beginning of the word to influence the meaning of the word root. Prefixes usually indicate the location, time, number, or status.
  - **Peri-** (meaning *around*) as in **pericardium**; the term *pericardium* refers to the membranous sac around the heart.
  - **Epi-** (meaning *above*) as in **epigastric**; the term *epigastric* describes the area above the stomach.

- Some prefixes can have opposing or contrasting meanings. For example, the prefix **intra-** means inside, the prefix **extra-**, outside.

Table 1.2 Contrasting Prefixes

Prefix	Contrasting Prefix
ab- to move away (from) *abduct* = to move away from the midline of the body	**ad-** to move toward *adduct* = to move toward the midline of the body
dys- abnormal, difficult *dyspnea* = difficult or labored breathing	**eu-** normal, good *euphoria* = a state of well being
hyper- excessive, above normal *hypertension* = high blood pressure	**hypo-** below normal *hypotension* = low blood pressure
pre- before *prenatal* = before birth	**post-** after *postmortem* = after death
tachy- fast *tachycardia* = fast heartbeat	**brady-** slow *bradycardia* = slow heartbeat

Suffixes

- A suffix is added to the end of the word root and usually indicates a **procedure, condition, disorder, or disease**. A suffix can totally change the meaning of a word root. For example, **megaly** (meaning enlargement) as in **cardiomegaly** (enlargement of the heart) and **algia** (meaning pain and suffering) as in **gastralgia** (stomach pain).
- **A suffix can make a word root a noun or an adjective**. For example, -um acts as a *noun ending* as in **cranium** and **ac** and –al act as *adjective endings* as in **cardiac** and **renal**.
- Many suffixes are related to specific disease conditions or pathology. **Path(o)** is the word root for *disease* and **–ology** is the suffix that means "*the study of*". Therefore, **pathology** is the *study of diseases*.

Table 1.3 Common Suffixes related to Disease Conditions and Procedures

Suffix	Meaning	Example(s)
-algia	pain	*neuralgia* = pain in the nerves
-centesis	surgical puncture	*abdominocentesis* = surgical puncture of the abdominal cavity to remove fluid
-ectomy	surgical removal	*tonsillectomy* = surgical removal of the tonsils
-itis	inflammation	*laryngitis* = inflammation of the larynx (voice box)
-lysis	destruction	*hemolysis* = destruction of red blood cells
-malacia	softening	*osteomalacia* = softening of the bone
-megaly	enlargement	*cardiomegaly* = enlargement of the heart
-necrosis	tissue death	*arterionecrosis* = tissue death of an artery or arteries

-otomy	cutting or surgical incision	*phlebotomy* = puncture of a vein for the purpose of drawing blood
-pathy	disease, suffering	*myopathy* = disease of the muscle
-ptosis	sagging or drooping	*blepharoptosis* = drooping of the upper eyelid

- Some suffixes begin with two letter "Rs." These suffixes are sometimes referred to the "**double RRs**." It is important to understand the differences among these suffixes.

Table 1.4 "Double R" Suffixes

Suffix	Meaning	Example(s)
-rrhage, -rrhagia	bleeding (sudden, severe flow)	*hemorrhage* = sudden, severe loss of blood
-rrhaphy	surgical suturing	*myorrhaphy* = surgical suturing of muscle
-rrhea	flow (of body fluids)	*amenorrhea* = absence of menstrual flow
-rrhexis	rupture	*myorrhexis* = rupture of muscle

Abbreviations, Acronyms, and Symbols

- **An abbreviation is a shortened form of a word or phrase.** For example, *Dr.* stands for Doctor and *epi* for epinephrine. An abbreviation is **also called a contraction or short form.**
- **An acronym is a word formed from the initial letters of other words; it is pronounced as a word.** For example, *AIDS* stands for Acquired Immune Deficiency Syndrome. Acronyms are sometimes incorrectly called abbreviations.
- **Symbols usually consist of one or more letters and/or numbers that represent an object, function, or process.** For example, in chemistry, the letter combination "*Na*" is the symbol for the element "sodium" (from Latin *natrium*).

Table 1.5 Examples of Abbreviations, Acronyms, and Symbols

Acronym/Abbreviation/Symbol	Meaning
BP	blood pressure
CNS	central nervous system
ECG, EKG	electrocardiogram
GYN	gynecology
ICU	intensive care unit
IM	intramuscular
IV	intravenous
KCl	potassium chloride
kg	kilogram

Eponyms, Antonyms, and Synonyms

- An **eponym** is a term or word based on or derived from a person's name. For example, **Lou Gehrig's disease** (or **amyotrophic lateral sclerosis**, **AML**) was named after an American baseball player who battled the disorder.
- **Antonyms** are words opposite in meaning to another. For example, **good** and **bad** are antonyms, as are long and short or wide and narrow.
- **Synonyms** are words or phrases that have exactly or nearly the same meaning as another word or phrase. For example, **shinbone** and **tibia** are synonyms, as are **thigh bone** and **femur**.
- A **thesaurus** is collection of words, terms, or phrases that have the same (synonyms) or opposite meaning (antonyms).

Plural Forms

- The **plural form** of most nouns is created simply by adding the letter 's'. However, there are a number of exceptions to this rule.

Table 1.6 Irregular Plural Forms

Singular	Example	Plural	Example
-a	vertebra	-ae	vertebrae
-is	diagnosis	-es	diagnoses
-en	lumen	-ina	lumina
-ma	stigma	-mata	stigmata
-on	phenomenon	-a	phenomena
-um	serum	-a	sera
-ex, -ix, -yx	index	-ices	indices
-nx	phalanx	-nges	phalanges
-us*	thrombus	-i	thrombi

* exceptions virus (viruses), sinus (sinuses), and plexus (plexuses)

Chapter 2 Basic Sciences Review

Carbohydrates, Lipids, and Proteins

- **Carbohydrates** contain three chemical elements: carbon (C), hydrogen (H), and oxygen (O). The basic formula is $C_nH_{2n}O_n$. For example, the formula form **glucose** is $C_6H_{12}O_6$.
  - Smaller carbohydrate molecules are called **sugars** because they taste sweet.
  - **Monosaccharides** (*mono*- one, *saccharide* sugar) or **simple sugars** consist of one unit only; **disaccharides** consist of two units, **trisaccharides** of three, and so on.
  - **Glucose** (aka **blood sugar** in medicine), **fructose** (**fruit sugar**), and **galactose** are the main monosaccharides of importance for our body. The three most common disaccharides are **sucrose** (aka **table sugar**, **cane sugar**, or **saccharose**), **lactose** (aka **milk sugar**), and **maltose** (aka **malt sugar**).
  - **Oligosaccharides** are usually formed from 3-10 monosaccharides, and **polysaccharides** can consist of long, linear chains or can be highly branched. Polysaccharides can be used as storage forms for carbohydrates in plants (**starch**) and animals (**glycogen**) as well as structural components, such as **cellulose** in plants and **chitin** in fungi and animals.

- **Lipids** do not dissolve in polar liquids, such as water, but rather in nonpolar liquids, such as acetone. They are mainly composed of carbon, hydrogen, and oxygen but may contain other elements, such as nitrogen and phosphorus.
  - The major lipids are **neutral fats** or **triglycerides**, **phospholipids**, **cholesterol**, and **eicosanoids**.
  - Each **triglyceride** consists of one molecule of **glycerol** and three molecules of **fatty acid**. Triglycerides are mainly used for energy storage and, to a lesser extent, as structural fat. They make up approximately 95% of all lipids of the human body.
  - Triglycerides can be subdivided into **saturated fats** that are found in meat, dairy products, and tropical oils (palm oil, coconut oil) and **unsaturated fats** from seeds, nuts, olive oil, and most other vegetable oils.
  - The **two essential fatty acids** (**linoleic acid** and **linolenic acid**) cannot be synthesized by our body and, therefore, must be ingested with food.
  - In **phospholipids** one fatty acid is replaced by a phosphate group, creating a molecule with a **hydrophilic** ("water-loving") **head** (the phosphate group) and a **hydrophobic** ("water-hating") **tail** (the two fatty acids).
  - Phospholipids are essential parts of the myelin sheaths of nerves and of the lipid bilayer cell membranes.
  - The **eicosanoids** contain **prostaglandins**, which have important functions such as smooth muscle contraction and blood pressure control, **thromboxanes**, and **leukotrienes**, which help regulate our immune system.
  - **Cholesterol** belongs to the **steroids**. It is a substantial part of animal cell membranes and a precursor of steroid hormones, e.g., sex hormones. Cholesterol is found in egg yolk, meats, shellfish, and milk products.

- **Proteins are made of amino acids.** There are 20 basic types of amino acids with different side chains. Two amino acids bound together form a **dipeptide**; three amino acids, a **tripeptide**; four amino acids, a **tetrapeptide** and so forth. **Polypeptides** consist of long chains of amino acids bound together by peptide bonds. When the chain contains more than 50 amino acids, the substance is called a **protein**.
  - The sequence of amino acids linked together is called the **primary structure** of the protein. The **secondary structure** results from folding of the protein chain. The

three-dimensional structure of a protein caused by the folding of the chain is called **tertiary structure**; it is important for the physical properties of the protein. Complex proteins consist of two or more individual protein chains or subunits, giving them a **quaternary structure** that is based on the spatial arrangement of the subunits.
- Proteins are used as **structural materials** for our body, for example, as keratin in skin and hair, but also play important roles as **functional proteins**, especially as **enzymes**.

Acids, Bases, and Electrolytes

- **Acids are proton donors**, i.e., substances that can give off (donate) protons or hydrogen ions (H^+); **bases are proton acceptors**. For example, HCl splits (dissociates) in water into protons (H^+) and chloride ions (Cl^-), thereby creating **hydrochloric acid**. **Sodium hydroxide** (NaOH) splits into sodium ions (Na^+) and hydroxide ions (^-OH). It is a base, because the hydroxide ions can accept protons to form water.
- **Strong acids and bases** dissociate (split up) completely in water; **weak acids and bases** only partially dissociate.
- When the concentration of hydrogen and hydroxide ions is the same, the solution is **neutral**; when there are more hydrogen ions than hydroxide ions, the solution is **acid-ic**; when there are fewer hydrogen ions than hydroxide ions, the solution is **alkaline** or **basic**.

- The **pH scale** is based on the H^+ concentration in the solution and **ranges from 0** (highest acidity) **to 14** (highest alkalinity). A **pH of 7 indicates a neutral solution**. As the **pH scale is a logarithmic scale**, a change in one unit for the pH represents a 10-fold increase or decrease in the H^+ concentration.

Figure 2.1 pH Scale

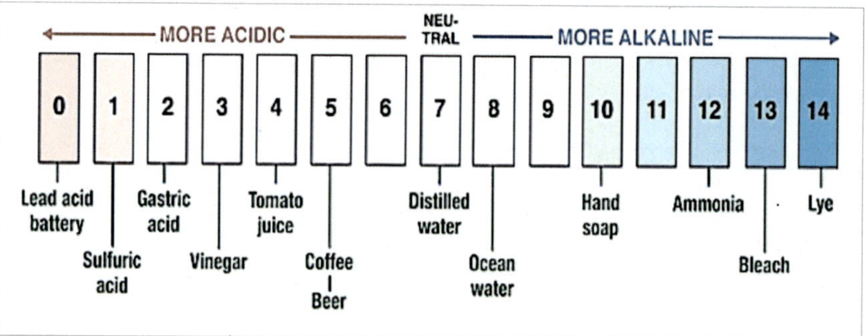

MORE ACIDIC						NEUTRAL			MORE ALKALINE				
0	1	2	3	4	5	6	7	8	9	10	11	12	13	14
Lead acid battery		Gastric acid		Tomato juice			Distilled water			Hand soap		Ammonia		Lye
	Sulfuric acid		Vinegar		Coffee / Beer				Ocean water				Bleach	

- **Electrolytes** are substances that dissociate into positive and negative ions in water; therefore, the watery solution will conduct electricity. Positively charged ions are called **cations**; negatively charged ions, **anions**.
- **Salts** are electrolytes that contain cations other than H^+, such as Na^+ (sodium) or K^+ (potassium). They are formed from the reaction between an acid and a base. For example, mixing hydrochloric acid (HCl) with sodium hydroxide (NaOH) generates **sodium chloride** (aka **table salt**) and water: $HCl + NaOH \rightarrow NaCl + H_2O$.
- Salts enter the human body by ingestion of food and drinks and are lost via perspiration, feces, and urine. They are important for controlling fluid movements, excitability of muscle and nerve cells, secretory activity, and membrane permeability.

Generalized Human Cell

- **Plasma membrane** - Flexible outer boundary; bimolecular layer of lipids and proteins in a constantly changing fluid mosaic; separates **intracellular fluid** (ICF) from **extracellular fluid** (ECF); ECF that surrounds cells = **interstitial fluid** (IF)
- **Cytoplasm** - Intracellular fluid containing organelles between plasma membrane and nucleus; consists of **cytosol** (water with solutes - (protein, salts, sugars, etc.), **cytoplasmic organelles** and **inclusions** (granules of glycogen or pigments, lipid droplets, vacuoles, and crystals)
- **Nucleus** - Control center containing **chromatin** (threadlike strands of DNA, histone proteins, and RNA); **nucleoli** are dark-staining spherical bodies involved in rRNA synthesis and ribosome subunit assembly; double-membrane **nuclear envelope** contains pores that regulate transport of large into and out of nucleus

Figure 2.2 Generalized Human Cell

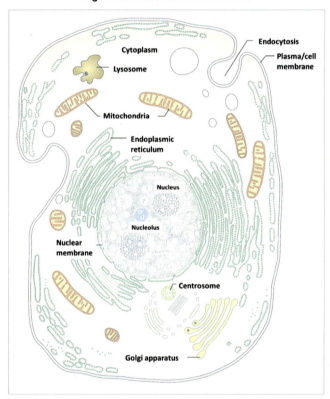

Cytoplasmic Organelles

Membranous Organelles
- **Mitochondria** - Double-membrane structure with shell-like cristae; contain their own DNA and RNA; provide most of cell's ATP via aerobic cellular respiration (powerhouse of the cell)
- **Endoplasmic Reticulum (ER)** - Interconnected tubes and parallel membranes en-

closing cisternae; continuous with nuclear membrane
- **Rough ER** - External surface studded with ribosomes; synthesizes all secreted proteins, membrane integral proteins and phospholipids
- **Smooth ER** - Tubules arranged in a looping network; enzyme function, e.g., lipid and cholesterol metabolism; synthesis of steroid hormones
- **Golgi Apparatus** - Stacked and flattened membranous sacs; modifies, concentrates, and packages proteins and lipids
- **Lysosomes** - Spherical membranous bags containing digestive enzymes (acid hydrolases); digest ingested bacteria, viruses, and toxins, nonfunctional organelles, injured or nonuseful tissue
- **Peroxisomes** - Membranous sacs containing powerful oxidases and catalases; detoxify harmful or toxic substances

Nonmembranous Organelles
- **Cytoskeleton**: Elaborate series of rods throughout cytosol
  - **Microfilaments** - actin strands involved in cell motility, change in shape, endocytosis and exocytosis
  - **Intermediate Filaments** - tough ropelike protein fibers; resist pulling forces on the cell and attach to desmosomes
  - **Microtubules** - Dynamic hollow tubes mostly radiating from centrosome
- **Ribosomes** - Granules containing protein and rRNA; site of protein synthesis; **free ribosomes** synthesize soluble proteins, **membrane-bound ribosomes** synthesize proteins to be incorporated into membranes or exported from the cell
- **Centrioles** - Small tubes formed by microtubules; part of centrosome

Plasma Membrane

- Bimolecular layer of lipids and proteins in a constantly changing fluid mosaic
- Plays a dynamic role in cellular activity
- Separates **intracellular fluid** (ICF) from **extracellular fluid** (ECF)
  - **Interstitial fluid** (IF) = ECF that surrounds cells
- **Membrane Lipids**
- 75% **phospholipids** (lipid bilayer)
  - **Phosphate heads**: polar and hydrophilic
  - **Fatty acid tails**: nonpolar and hydrophobic
- 5% **glycolipids** - Lipids with polar sugar groups on outer membrane surface
- 20% **cholesterol** - Increases membrane stability and fluidity
- **Lipid Rafts**
- ~ 20% of the outer membrane surface; contain phospholipids, sphingolipids, and cholesterol; may function as stable platforms for cell-signaling molecules
- **Membrane Proteins**
- **Integral proteins** - Firmly inserted into the membrane (most are transmembrane)
  - *Functions*: Transport proteins (channels and carriers), enzymes, or receptors
- **Peripheral proteins** - Loosely attached to integral proteins. Include filaments on intracellular surface and glycoproteins on extracellular surface
  - *Functions*: Enzymes, motor proteins, cell-to-cell links, support on intracellular surface, glycocalyx

Membrane Junctions

- **Tight junctions**: Prevent fluids and most molecules from moving between cells
- **Desmosomes**: Rivets" or "spot-welds" that anchor cells together
- **Gap junctions**: Transmembrane proteins form pores that allow small molecules to pass from cell to cell. For spread of ions between cardiac or smooth muscle cells

Cellular Extensions

- **Cilia** are whip-like, motile cellular extensions on the exposed apical surfaces of some cells that move substances across cell surfaces.
- **Flagella** are long cellular projections that move the cell through the environment, e.g., the tail of the sperm.
- **Microvilli** are finger-like extensions of the plasma membrane that increase the surface area of a cell, e.g., for absorption.

Transport Processes across Membranes

	Simple Diffusion: Nonpolar lipid-soluble (hydrophobic) substances diffuse directly through the phospholipid bilayer
	Facilitated Diffusion: Some molecules (e.g., glucose, amino acids, and ions) use carrier or channel proteins; exhibits specificity (selectivity); is saturable (rate is determined by number of carriers/channels); can be regulated in terms of activity and quantity
Passive processes - No cellular energy (ATP) required; substance moves down its concentration gradient	• **Carrier proteins** - transmembrane integral proteins transport specific polar molecules (e.g., sugars and amino acids); binding of substrate causes shape change in carrier • **Channel proteins** - aqueous channels formed by transmembrane proteins; selectively transport ions or water; **leakage channels** always open - **gated channels** controlled by chemical or electrical signals
	Osmosis: Movement of solvent (water) across a selectively permeable membrane; water enters or leaves a cell • **Osmolarity** = number of solutes in 1 liter of solution [osmol/l or Osm/l] • **Osmolality** = number of solutes in 1 kg of solvent [osmol/kg or Osm/kg] • **Isotonic solution** - same solute concentration as cytosol • **Hypertonic solution** - greater solute concentration than cytosol • **Hypotonic solution** - lesser solute concentration than cytosol
Movement caused by a pressure gradient	**Filtration**: Movement of a solution across a permeable membrane.
	Primary Active Transport: Energy from hydrolysis of ATP is used to pump solute (ions) across the membrane • **Sodium-potassium pump** (Na^+-K^+ ATPase) located in all plasma membranes; involved in primary and secondary active transport of nutrients and ions Maintains electrochemical gradients essential for functions of muscle and nerve

Active processes - Energy (ATP) and carrier proteins (solute pumps) required; moves solutes against a concentration gradient	tissues

	Secondary Active Transport: Depends on an ion gradient created by primary active transport; energy stored in gradients is used to drive transport of other solutes
	• **Cotransport** - always transports more than one substance at a time
	  • **Symport** system: Two substances transported in same direction
	  • **Antiport** system: Two substances transported in opposite directions

	Vesicular Transport of large particles, macromolecules, and fluids across plasma membranes • **Exocytosis** - transport out of cell • **Endocytosis** - transport into cell • **Transcytosis** - transport into, across, and then out of cell • **Substance (vesicular) trafficking** - transport from one area or organelle in cell to another

Tonicity

The ability of a solution to cause water to flow into the cell or to flow out of the cell.
- **Isotonic solutions** have the same solute concentration as that of the cytosol. Thus, no osmosis will occur.
- **Hypertonic solutions** have a greater solute concentration than the cytosol. Water will move out leading to shrinkage of the cell.
- **Hypotonic solutions** have a lesser solute concentration than the cytosol. Water moves into the cell causing swelling and, eventually, cell lysis.

Resting Membrane Potential & Action Potential

Resting Membrane Potential
- **Potential difference across the membrane of a resting cell**
- **Generated by:**
  - **Differences in ionic makeup of ICF and ECF**
    - ICF has lower concentration of Na^+ and Cl^- than ECF
    - ICF has higher concentration of K^+ and negatively charged proteins (A^-) than ECF
  - **Differential permeability of the plasma membrane**
    - Impermeable to A^-, freely permeable to Cl^-
    - Slightly permeable to Na^+ (through leakage channels)
    - 75 times more permeable to K^+ (more leakage channels)
- **Negative interior of the cell due to much greater diffusion of K^+ out of the cell than Na^+ diffusion into the cell**
- **Sodium-potassium pump** stabilizes the resting membrane potential by maintaining the concentration gradients for Na^+ and K^+

Proteins serve as **two main types of membrane ion channels**:
- **Leakage (nongated) channels** - always open
- **Gated channels** (three types):
  - **Chemically gated** (ligand-gated) **channels** - open with binding of a specific neuro-

transmitter
- **Voltage-gated channels** - open and close in response to changes in membrane potential
- **Mechanically gated channels** - open and close in response to physical deformation of receptors
- When gated channels are open:
  - Ions diffuse quickly across the membrane along their electrochemical gradients
  - Along chemical concentration gradients from higher concentration to lower concentration
  - Along electrical gradients toward opposite electrical charge
  - Ion flow creates an electrical current and voltage changes across the membrane

Changes in membrane potential are signals used to receive, integrate and send information.
- Membrane potential changes when concentrations of ions across the membrane change and/or permeability of membrane to ions changes
- **Depolarization**: A reduction in membrane potential (toward zero) → inside of the membrane less negative → increases the probability of producing a nerve impulse
- **Hyperpolarization**: An increase in membrane potential (away from zero) → inside of the membrane more negative → reduces the probability of producing a nerve impulse

Graded Potentials - Short-lived, localized changes in membrane potential
- Spread as local currents change the membrane potential of adjacent regions
- Occur when a stimulus causes gated ion channels to open
- Magnitude varies directly (graded) with stimulus strength
- Decrease in magnitude with distance as ions diffuse through leakage channels
- Short-distance signals

- **Properties of gated Na^+ and K^+ channels**
  - Each **Na^+ channel** has two voltage-sensitive gates
    - Activation gate: **Closed at rest; open with depolarization**
    - Inactivation gate: **Open at rest; block channel once it is open**
  - Each **K^+ channel** has one voltage-sensitive gate
    - Closed at rest
    - Opens slowly with depolarization

Action Potential (AP) - Brief reversal of membrane potential with a total amplitude of ~100 mV
- Does not decrease in magnitude over distance
- Principal means of long-distance neural communication
- **AP is an all-or-none phenomenon** - action potentials either happen completely, or not at all
- All action potentials are alike and are independent of stimulus intensity
- Strong stimuli can generate action potentials more often than weaker stimuli
- The CNS determines stimulus intensity by the frequency of impulses

- **Generation of an Action Potential**
  - **Resting state [1]**: Only leakage channels for Na^+ and K^+ are open; all gated Na^+ and K^+ channels are closed
  - **Depolarizing Phase [2]**: Depolarizing local currents open voltage-gated Na^+ chan-

nels → Na^+ influx causes more depolarization → at threshold (−55 to −50 mV) positive feedback leads to opening of all Na^+ channels, and a reversal of membrane polarity to +30mV (spike of action potential)
- **Repolarizing Phase [3]**: Na^+ channel slow inactivation gates close → membrane permeability to Na^+ declines to resting levels; slow voltage-sensitive K^+ gates open → K^+ exits the cell and internal negativity is restored
- **Hyperpolarization [4]**: Some K^+ channels remain open, allowing excessive K^+ efflux → after-hyperpolarization of the membrane (undershoot)
- **Role of the Sodium-Potassium Pump**
  - Repolarization restores the resting electrical conditions of the neuron, but does not restore the resting ionic conditions
  - Ionic redistribution back to resting conditions is restored by of Na+-K+ pumps
- **Propagation of an Action Potential**
  - Na^+ influx causes a patch of the axonal membrane to depolarize; local currents occur → affect adjacent areas in the forward direction → depolarization opens voltage-gated channels and triggers an AP
  - Repolarization wave follows the depolarization wave
  - At **threshold**: Membrane is depolarized by 15 to 20 mV → Na^+ permeability increases → Na influx exceeds K^+ efflux → positive feedback cycle begins
- **Absolute Refractory Period**: Time from the opening of the Na^+ channels until the resetting of the channels; ensures that each AP is an all-or-none event; enforces one-way transmission of nerve impulses
- **Relative Refractory Period**: Follows the absolute refractory period; repolarization is occurring; threshold for AP generation is elevated; exceptionally strong stimulus may generate an AP

Figure 2.2 Action Potential

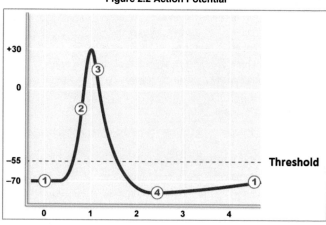

A&P Essentials 4th ed.

Chapter 3 Introduction into Anatomy & Physiology

Overview of Anatomy and Physiology

Anatomy: The study of structure
- **Gross** or **macroscopic anatomy studies** structures visible with the unaided eye, **microscopic anatomy**, structures visible under a microscope only
- **Surface anatomy** studies the surface of the body as well as structures that are visible underneath the surface, such as the kneecaps
- **Systemic anatomy** subdivides the body into systems, such as the cardiovascular system (**cardiovascular anatomy**)
- **Regional** or **topographical anatomy** focuses on the interaction of different systemic structures in a defined region of the body, such as the shoulder or hip
- **Developmental anatomy** looks at how our body evolved and developed over time or during our time from conception to birth (**embryology**)
- **Cytology** is the study of cells; **histology** is the study of tissues
- **The principal tool for the study of anatomy is mastery of anatomical terminology**

Physiology: The study of function of the whole body or its systems and organs on many levels
- Subdivided into the physiology of organs (e.g., **renal physiology**) and systems (e.g., **cardiovascular physiology**).
- **Essential tools** for the study of physiology are an ability to focus on different levels (from systemic to cellular and molecular) and knowledge of basic principles of biology, physics, and chemistry.

Principle of Complementarity: Anatomy and physiology are inseparable; function always reflects structure; what a structure can do depends on its specific form

Figure 3.1 Surface anatomy of the back and front of body

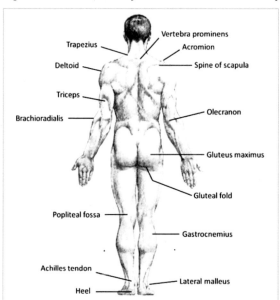

13

A&P Essentials 4th ed.

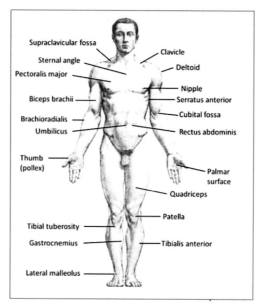

Six levels of Structural Organization

• **Chemical**: atoms and molecules
• **Cellular**: cells and their organelles
• **Tissue**: groups of similar cells
• **Organ**: contains two or more types of tissues
• **Organ system**: organs that work closely together
• **Organismal**: all organ systems

Organs & Organ Systems

Organs are structures that **are made of two or more tissues.**
The **eleven organ systems** in the human body have to work together to keep the body healthy as all cells depend on them to meet their survival needs.
1. **Integumentary System**: External body covering; protects deeper tissues from injury; synthesizes vitamin D; pain, pressure, etc. receptors; sweat and oil glands.
2. **Skeletal System**: Protects and supports body organs; provides framework for muscles to attach to; site of blood cell formation; stores minerals.
3. **Muscular System**: Allows manipulation of the environment, locomotion, and facial expression; maintains posture; produces heat.
4. **Nervous System**: Fast-acting control system of the body; responds to internal and external changes by activating muscles and glands.
5. **Endocrine System**: Secretes hormones for growth, reproduction, and nutrient use (metabolism) by body cells.
6. **Cardiovascular System**: Pumps/transports blood, which carries oxygen, carbon dioxide, nutrients, wastes, etc.

7. **Lymphatic System/Immunity**: Picks up fluid leaked from blood vessels and returns it to blood; disposes of debris in the lymphatic stream; backbone of the immune system.
8. **Respiratory System**: Keeps blood constantly supplied with oxygen and removes carbon dioxide.
9. **Digestive System**: Breaks down food and absorbs nutrients; indigestible foodstuffs are eliminated as feces.
10. **Urinary System**: Eliminates nitrogenous wastes from the body; regulates water, electrolyte and acid-base balance of the blood.
11. **Reproductive System**: Production of offspring; gonads (testes, ovaries) produce sperm/eggs and sex hormones; ducts and glands aid in delivery of sperm to the female reproductive tract; female structures serve as sites for fertilization and development of the fetus; mammary glands produce milk to nourish the newborn.

Homeostasis

Maintenance of a relatively stable internal environment despite continuous outside changes; a dynamic state of equilibrium.

- Homeostatic control mechanisms involve continuous monitoring and regulation of many factors (variables)

- In a **control mechanism,** the **receptor/sensor** monitors sends input signals to the **control center**, which compares the signal to a record of the set point at which the variable is to be maintained. If it determines that action is required it sends instructions to the **effector**, which responds by reducing or enhancing the original stimulus. The whole system is called a **feedback mechanism**.
  - **Negative Feedback**: The response reduces or shuts off the original stimulus.(99% of all feedback mechanisms)
  - **Positive Feedback**: The response enhances or exaggerates the original stimulus

Eight Necessary Life Functions

Are essential for keeping our body and mind healthy. **If one or more of them cannot be maintained properly, signs and symptoms of disease will develop**.
1. Maintaining boundaries between internal and external environments
2. Movement (contractility)
3. Responsiveness (ability to sense and respond to stimuli)
4. Digestion
5. Metabolism
6. Excretion
7. Reproduction
8. Growth

Five Survival Needs

Must be met at all times or the body will suffer and may die.
1. Nutrients
2. Oxygen
3. Water
4. Normal body temperature

5. Appropriate atmospheric pressure

Nutrients

Nutrient: a substance in food that promotes normal growth, maintenance, and repair
- **Major nutrients**: Carbohydrates, lipids, and proteins
- **Other nutrients**: Vitamins and minerals (and water)

Carbohydrates
- **Dietary sources: Starch** (complex carbohydrates) in grains and vegetables; **sugars** in fruits, sugarcane, sugar beets, honey and milk
- **Uses: Glucose** used by cells to make ATP (4 kcal per gram); **insoluble fiber**: cellulose in vegetables; provides roughage; **soluble fiber**: pectin in apples and citrus fruits; reduces blood cholesterol levels
- **Dietary requirements: Recommended intake**: 45–65% of total calorie intake; mostly complex carbohydrates; **minimum** 100 g/day to maintain adequate blood glucose levels

Proteins
- **Dietary sources:** Eggs, milk, fish, and most meats contain complete proteins; legumes, nuts, and cereals contain incomplete protein, but together contain all essential amino acids
- **Uses: Structural proteins**: keratin, collagen, elastin, muscle proteins; **functional proteins**: enzymes, some hormones; used as fuel if insufficient carbohydrate or fat available (4 kcal per gram)
- **Dietary requirements: Rule of thumb**: daily intake of 0.8 g per kg body weight = 1 egg; **All-or-none rule**: All amino acids must be present for protein synthesis to occur

Lipids
- **Dietary sources: Saturated fats** in meat, dairy foods, and tropical oils; **unsaturated fats** in seeds, nuts, olive oil, and most vegetable oils; **cholesterol** in egg yolk, meats, organ meats, shellfish, and milk products
- **Uses: Major fuel** of hepatocytes and skeletal muscle (9 kcal per gram); help **absorb fat-soluble vitamins**; **phospholipids** are essential in myelin sheaths and all cell membranes; **adipose tissue** forms around body organs and insulating layer below skin; concentrated source of energy; **cholesterol** stabilizes membranes and is a precursor of bile salts and steroid hormones
- **Dietary requirements:** Fats should represent **30% or less of total caloric intake**; **saturated fats** should be limited to 10% or less of total fat intake; daily **cholesterol** intake should be **no more than 300 mg**; **essential fatty acids** (linoleic and linolenic) acid, found in most vegetable oils

Vitamins
- Organic compounds; most function as coenzymes; crucial in helping the body use nutrients
- Vitamins D, some B, and K are synthesized in the body
  - **Water-soluble vitamins** - B complex and C are absorbed with water B_{12} absorption requires intrinsic factor; not stored in the body
  - **Fat-soluble vitamins** - A, D, E, and K are absorbed with lipid digestion products; stored in the body, except for vitamin K

Minerals
- Work with nutrients to ensure proper body functioning

- Uptake and excretion must be balanced to prevent toxic overload
- Required in moderate (calcium, phosphorus, potassium, sulfur, sodium, chloride, magnesium, iron in women) or trace amounts (e.g., iron, in men, zinc, manganese, iodine)

Energy Balance

- **Energy intake** = the energy liberated during food oxidation
- **Energy output**
  - Immediately lost as heat (~60%)
  - Used to do work (driven by ATP)
- **Energy intake has to equal the total energy output**

Quetelet index or **Body mass index** (BMI) = wt (lb) × 705/ht (inches)^2
- **Underweight**: < 18.5
- **Normal weight**: 18.5 – 24.9
- **Overweight**: 25 – 29.9
- **Obesity**: ≥ 30; the **World Health Organization** (WHO) further breaks down obesity into three classes:
  - **Class I: Obesity** (BMI 30.0 – 34.9)
  - **Class II: Severe Obesity** (BMI 35.0 – 39.9)
  - **Class III: Morbid Obesity** (BMI ≥ 40)
- Higher incidence of atherosclerosis, diabetes mellitus, hypertension, heart disease, and osteoarthritis among overweight and, especially, obese people
- **BMI does not account for the composition of the body**. Muscle and fat tissue have the same weight and are considered equal as far as BMI is concerned

Body fat falls into two categories, **essential** (or **structural**) **fat** and **storage fat**.
- **Essential fat** is needed for normal physiological function. Men have about 3% essential fat (of the total body weight), women 12% (more fat in breasts and uterus, less muscles mass).
- **Storage fat** is stored in adipose tissue around major organs and in the peritoneal cavity and approx. 50% as subcutaneous fat beneath the skin. Women store fat more around hips and thighs (**pear shape**), men around the waist (**apple shape**).

Oxygen

A sufficient **oxygen** supply at any given time is essential for all human cells, tissues, and organs.
- **Hypoxia**: Oxygen supply is not meeting demands and a situation of low oxygen level in the tissues develops
- **Anoxia**: no oxygen available at all
- **Hypoxemia**: Hypoxia caused by low oxygen level in the blood
- **Ischemia**: Hypoxia caused by poor blood flow (perfusion)

Severe hypoxia will lead to cell death (necrosis) in the affected area.
- If the necrosis is caused by poor blood flow (**ischemia**), the area with necrotic tissue is called an **infarct** and the whole mechanism, an **infarction**.

Water

Water is the most abundant chemical in the body and site of chemical reactions.

- Our **body water content depends on our age and gender**.
  - **Infants**: 73% or more water (low body fat, low bone mass)
  - **Adult males**: ~60% water
  - **Adult females**: ~50% water (higher fat content, less skeletal muscle mass)
  - Water content declines to ~45% in old age

When the output (water loss) exceeds water intake, a **negative fluid balance** develops and we become **dehydrated**.
- Water loss may be due to hemorrhage, severe burns, prolonged vomiting or diarrhea, profuse sweating, water deprivation, and diuretic abuse.
- Symptoms are thirst, dry, flushed skin, and low urine production (oliguria).
- It may lead to weight loss, fever, mental confusion, and hypovolemic shock (see also **Chapter 23 Fluid, Electrolyte, and Acid-Base Balance**)

Body Temperature

Body temperature reflects the balance between heat production and heat loss
- At rest, the liver, heart, brain, kidneys, and endocrine organs generate most heat
- **Normal body temperature** = 98.6°F
- Organs in the core have the highest temperature
  - Women have a slightly higher core temperature (97.8°F) than men (97.4°F) but colder hands (87.2°F) compared to men (90°F).
- Blood is the major agent of heat exchange between the core and the shell
- **Core temperature** is regulated and remains relatively constant, **shell temperature** fluctuates substantially (68-104°F)

Mechanisms of Heat Exchange
- **Radiation** is the loss of heat in the form of infrared rays
- **Conduction** is the transfer of heat by direct contact
- **Convection** is the transfer of heat to the surrounding air
- **Evaporation** is the heat loss due to the evaporation of water from body surfaces
  - **Insensible heat loss** accompanies **insensible water loss** from lungs, oral mucosa, and skin
  - **Evaporative heat loss** becomes **sensible** (active) when body temperature rises and sweating increases water vaporization

The **hypothalamus** has **two thermoregulatory centers**, one **heat-loss center** and one **heat-promoting center**
- **Hyperthermia** - Elevated body temperature depresses the hypothalamus
  - Positive-feedback mechanism (heat stroke) begins at core temperature of 41°C (106°F)
  - Can be fatal if not corrected
- **Heat exhaustion** - Heat-associated collapse after vigorous activity
  - Due to dehydration and low blood pressure
  - Heat-loss mechanisms are still functional
  - May progress to heat stroke
- **Hypothermia** - Low body temperature where vital signs decrease
  - Shivering stops at core temperature of 30-32°C (86-90°F)
  - Can progress to coma a death by cardiac arrest at ~ 21°C (70°F)

A&P Essentials 4th ed.

Appropriate Atmospheric Pressure

Vital for adequate breathing and gas exchange in the lungs
* Quick travel to altitudes above 8000 feet may produce symptoms of **acute mountain sickness** (AMS) such as headaches, shortness of breath, nausea, and dizziness; in severe cases, lethal cerebral and pulmonary edema
* **Acclimatization**: respiratory and hematopoietic long-term adjustments to altitude
* Decline in blood O_2 causes kidneys to increase **erythropoietin** (EPO) release
* EPO travels to the red bone marrow and causes the formation and release of new red blood cells into the blood
* Having more red blood cells allows the blood to take in and transport more oxygen

Regional and Directional Terms

* **Regional terms** designate specific areas, i.e., they are adjectives relating to a defined structure
* **Directional terms** describe the location of a structure in relation to other structures or locations
* Some terms, such as cranial, can be used as either regional or directional term
* **Directional terms are always based on the standard anatomical position**

Table 3.1 Examples of Regional and Directional Terms

Regional term	Definition	Directional term	Definition
abdominal	relating to the abdomen	**anterior**	closer to the front of the body
brachial	relating to the arm	**contralateral**	on opposite sides of the body
cervical	relating to a neck or cervix	**cranial**	toward the head
cranial	relating to the cranium or skull	**deep**	farther away from the surface of the body
femoral	relating to the femur	**distal**	farther away from the body
humeral	relating to the upper arm or humerus	**inferior**	below, lower
lumbar	relating to the loins	**ipsilateral**	on the same side of the body
malleolar	relating to ankle/malleolus or ankle region	**lateral**	away from the midline of the body
nasal	relating to the nose	**medial**	toward the midline of the body
pelvic	relating to the pelvis	**posterior**	closer to the back of the body
radial	relating to the radius	**proximal**	nearer/closer to the body
spinal	relating to the spine or	**superficial**	close(r) to the surface

	the spinal cord		
thoracic	relating to the thorax or chest region	**superior**	above; higher

Standard Anatomical Position & Body Planes

The **standard anatomical position** describes the body in a standing upright position with the hands turned out so that the palms are facing forward. Anatomists and clinicians use this standard position to describe the location of organs or body parts to each other.

Body planes are flat surfaces along which the body or a structure is cut for anatomical or pathological study. Any diagonal cut, regardless of the plane it lies in, produces an **oblique section**.
- **Sagittal plane** divides body vertically into right and left parts □ sagittal section
  - **Midsagittal (median) plane**: Lies on midline
  - **Parasagittal plane**: Not on midline
- **Frontal (coronal) plane** divides body vertically into anterior and posterior parts
- **Transverse (horizontal) plane** Divides body horizontally into superior and inferior parts → cross section
- **Oblique section** runs diagonally

Figure 3.2 Standard anatomical position (left) and body planes (right)

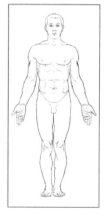
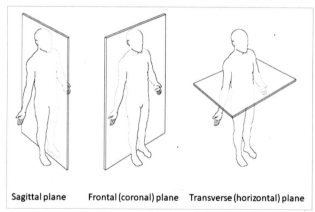

Sagittal plane   Frontal (coronal) plane   Transverse (horizontal) plane

Body Cavities

Dorsal cavity – protects the nervous system	• **Cranial cavity** encases the brain • **Vertebral cavity** encases the spinal cord

Ventral cavity - houses internal organs (viscera)	• **Thoracic cavity**
	  • Two **pleural cavities** house the lung
	  • **Mediastinum** contains **pericardial cavity**, which encloses heart
	• **Abdominopelvic cavity**
	  • **Abdominal cavity** contains stomach, intestines, spleen, and liver

	• **Pelvic cavity** contains urinary bladder, reproductive organs, and rectum

Figure 3.3 Body cavities

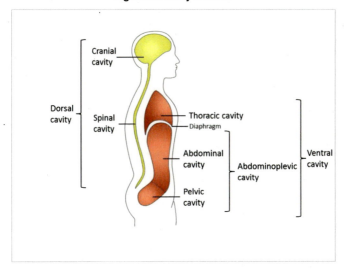

Figure 3.4 Abdominopelvic regions (left) and quadrants (right)

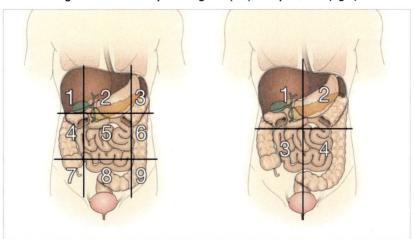

Abdominopelvic Regions and Quadrants (numbers refer to figure 3.4)

Abdominopelvic Regions
- Right and left hypochondriac region (1, 3)
- Epigastric region (2)
- Right and left lumbar region (4, 6)
- Umbilical region (5)
- Right and left iliac/inguinal region (7, 9)

- Hypogastric/pubic region (8)

Abdominopelvic Quadrants
- Right and left upper quadrant (1, 2)
- Right and left lower quadrant (3, 4)

Figure 3.5 Abdominopelvic regions (left) and quadrants (right) and major organs

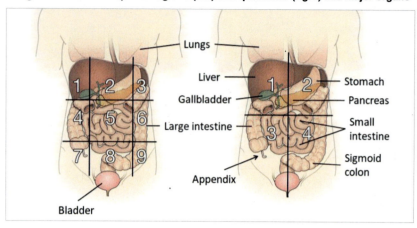

A&P Essentials 4th ed.

Chapter 4 Histology

- **Tissue** - Groups of cells similar in structure and function
- Four **basic types of tissue**
  - Epithelial tissue
  - Connective tissue
  - Nervous tissue
  - Muscle tissue

Epithelial Tissue (Epithelium)

- Two main types (by location):
  - **Covering and lining epithelia** - on external and internal surfaces
  - **Glandular epithelia** – the secretory tissue in glands
- **Cells have polarity** - apical (upper, free) and basal (lower, attached) surfaces; continuous sheets of closely packed cells held together by tight junctions and desmosomes
- **Noncellular basal lamina** of glycoprotein and collagen lies adjacent to basal surface supported by a connective tissue reticular lamina
- Avascular but innervated; high rate of regeneration

Classification of Epithelia

- 1 layer of cells = simple epithelium; >1 = stratified epithelium
- Squamous, cuboidal or columnar depending on (apical) layer of cells
- **Simple squamous epithelium** - Single layer of flattened cells with disc-shaped central nuclei and sparse cytoplasm; **endothelium** (heart, vessels); **mesothelium**
- **Simple cuboidal epithelium** - Single layer of cube-like cells with large, spherical central nuclei
- **Simple columnar epithelium** - Single layer of tall cells with round to oval nuclei; some cells bear cilia; may contain mucus-secreting goblet cells
- **Pseudostratified columnar epithelium** - Single layer of cells of differing heights, some not reaching the free surface; nuclei seen at different levels; may contain mucus-secreting goblet cells and bear cilia
- **Stratified squamous epithelium** - Composed of several cell layers; basal cells are cuboidal or columnar, surface cells are flattened (squamous); in the keratinized type, the surface cells are full of keratin and dead
- **Stratified cuboidal epithelium** - Typically two cell layers thick; rare
- **Stratified columnar epithelium** - Limited distribution in body
- **Transitional epithelium** - Resembles both stratified squamous and stratified cuboidal; basal cells cuboidal or columnar; surface cells dome shaped or squamous-like

Glandular Epithelia

Gland = one or more cells that makes and secretes an (aqueous) fluid

- Classified by:
  - Number of cells forming the gland - **unicellular** (e.g., goblet cells) or **multicellular**

- **Presence or absence of duct system:**
  - **Endocrine** (ductless) **glands** secrete hormones that travel through lymph or blood to target organs
  - **Exocrine glands** secrete products via ducts onto body surfaces (skin) or into body cavities
  - The only important **unicellular exocrine gland** is the goblet cell
  - **Multicellular exocrine glands** are composed of a duct and a secretory unit; classifies by duct type (simple vs. compound) and structure of secretory units (tubular, alveolar, or tubuloalveolar)
- **Modes of Secretion**
  - **Merocrine** - Products are secreted by exocytosis (e.g., pancreas, sweat and salivary glands)
  - **Holocrine** - Products are secreted by rupture of gland cells (e.g., sebaceous glands)

Epithelial Membranes

- **Cutaneous membrane (skin)** – see Chapter 4 Integumentary System

- **Mucous membranes (Mucosae)** - Line body cavities open to the exterior (e.g., digestive and respiratory tracts)

- **Serous Membranes (Serosae)** - Line closed cavities; consist of epithelium plus underlying areolar tissue
  - **Parietal serosae** line internal body walls
  - **Visceral serosae** cover internal organs
  - Separated by (virtual) **cavity** containing fluid to reduce friction

Connective Tissues

- Four classes
  - Connective tissue proper
  - Cartilage
  - Bone tissue
  - Blood

- Connective tissues have:
  - **Cells** separated by nonliving **extracellular matrix** (ground substance and fibers)
  - Varying degrees of vascularity

- **Cells**: Mitotically active and secretory cells = "**blasts**"; mature cells = "**cytes**"
  - **Fibroblasts** and **fibrocytes** in **connective tissue proper**
  - **Chondroblasts** and **chondrocytes** in **cartilage**
  - **Osteoblasts** and **osteocytes** in **bone**
  - **Hematopoietic stem cells** in **bone marrow**
  - Fat cells, white blood cells, mast cells, and macrophages

- **Ground substance**: Medium through which solutes diffuse between blood capillaries and cells; consists of interstitial fluid, adhesion proteins, proteoglycans

- **Three types of fibers**
  - **Collagen** (white fibers): Strongest and most abundant type; provides high tensile strength

- **Elastic**: Networks of long, thin, elastin fibers that allow for stretch
- **Reticular**: Short, fine, highly branched collagenous fibers

Classification of Connective Tissues Proper

- Loose connective tissue
  - Areolar
  - Adipose
  - Reticular
- Dense connective tissue
  - Regular
  - Irregular
  - Elastic

- **Areolar loose connective tissue** - Gel-like matrix with all three fiber type, fibroblasts, macrophages, mast cells, and some white blood cells; widely distributed under epithelia of body, packages organs; surrounds capillaries

- **Adipose loose connective tissue** - Closely packed adipocytes (fat cells); provides reserve food fuel; insulates against heat loss (under skin); supports and protects organs (kidneys and eyeballs; abdomen; breasts)

- **Reticular loose connective tissue** - Network of reticular fibers in a typical loose ground substance; reticular cells lie on the network; forms soft internal skeleton (stroma) of lymph nodes, bone marrow, and spleen

- **Dense regular connective tissue** – Mostly parallel collagen fibers; a few elastic fibers; withstands great tensile stress when pulling force is applied in one direction; in tendons, ligaments, aponeuroses

- **Dense irregular connective tissue** - Primarily irregularly arranged collagen fibers; some elastic fibers; withstands tension exerted in many directions; provides structural strength; fibrous capsules of organs and of joints; dermis of the skin; submucosa of digestive tract

- **Elastic connective tissue** - Contain a high proportion of elastic fibers; allows recoil of tissue following stretching (arteries, lung)

Cartilage

- **Hyaline Cartilage** - Amorphous but firm matrix; collagen fibers form an imperceptible network; chondroblasts produce the matrix and when mature (chondrocytes) lie in lacunae; supports and reinforces; has resilient cushioning properties; resists compressive stress; forms most of the embryonic skeleton; covers the ends of long bones in joint cavities; forms costal cartilages of the ribs, cartilages of the nose, trachea, and larynx

- **Elastic Cartilage** - Similar to hyaline cartilage, but more elastic fibers in matrix; flexible with shape memory; found in external ear (pinna), epiglottis, and Eustachian tube

- **Fibrocartilage** - Similar to hyaline cartilage, but abundance of thick collagen fibers give it tensile strength with the ability to absorb compressive shock; found in intervertebral discs, pubic symphysis, and menisci of knee joint

Bone (osseous) Tissue (see Chapter 6 Bones & Skeletal Tissues)

- Hard, calcified matrix containing many collagen fibers. Mature osteocytes lie in lacunae. Bone tissue is very well vascularized.

Blood (see Chapter 18 Blood, Hemostasis, and Blood Groups)

- Consists of cells (red & white blood cells) surrounded by a liquid matrix (plasma).

Nervous Tissue (see Chapter 11 Nervous Tissue)

- Has two groups of cells:
  - **Neurons** (nerve cells) are excitable cells that form the major active parts of the nervous system.
  - **Neuroglia** are non-excitable supporting cells.

Muscle Tissue (see Chapter 9 Muscle Tissue)

- There are three types of muscle tissues:
  - **Smooth muscle**: Spindle-shaped cells with central nuclei; no striations; involuntary; can generate its own contraction rhythm.
  - **Cardiac muscle**: Found in the heart only; branching, striated, usually uninucleate cells; involuntary and can generate its own contraction rhythm.
  - **Skeletal muscle**: Long, cylindrical cells with many nuclei and striations; voluntary; attaches to bones or skin.

Tissue Repair

- **Regeneration**: Damaged cells are replaced with the same type of cell and the original function of the tissue is restored.
- **Fibrosis**: Damaged cells are replaced with fibrous connective tissue creating scar tissue.
  - **Step 1**: Inflammatory response prepares the damaged area for the repair. Formation of a blood clot (scab).
  - **Step 2**: Restoration of blood supply. Blood clot replaced with granulation tissue. Epithelium begins to regenerate.
  - **Step 3**: Regeneration and fibrosis. Scab detaches. Regenerated epithelium with underlying scar tissue.
- **Different tissues have different regenerative capacities**:
  - Epithelial tissues, bone tissue, areolar connective tissue, dense irregular connective tissue, and blood-forming tissue regenerate extremely well.
  - Smooth muscle and dense regular connective tissue have moderate regenerating capacities.
  - Cardiac muscle and the nervous tissue of brain and spinal cord are amitotic and have more or less no functional regenerative capacity.

Chapter 5 Integumentary System

Skin (Integument) (numbers refer to figure 5.1)

Epidermis - superficial region **[A]**
- Upper, avascular keratinized stratified squamous epithelium
- Cells of epidermis
  - **Keratinocytes** - produce fibrous protein **keratin**
  - **Melanocytes** - 10–25% of cells in lower epidermis; produce pigment **melanin**
  - **Epidermal dendritic (Langerhans) cells** - macrophages that help activate immune system
  - **Tactile (Merkel) cells** - touch receptors

Stratum Corneum (Horny Layer) [1]	• Uppermost layer; 20–30 rows of dead, flat, keratinized membranous sacs; ¾ of epidermis; protects from abrasion and penetration, biological, chemical, and physical assaults; waterproofs
Stratum Lucidum (Clear Layer) [2]	• In thick skin (palm, sole) only; thin, transparent band; a few rows of flat, dead keratinocytes
Stratum Granulosum (Granular Layer) [3]	• Thin (3-5 cells) layer in which the cells flatten; keratohyaline and lamellated granules accumulate
Stratum Spinosum (Prickly Layer) [4]	• Cells contain a web-like system of intermediate prekeratin filaments attached to desmosomes; lots of melanin granules and dendritic cells
Stratum Basale (Basal Layer) [5]	• Single row of stem cells; firmly attached to basal lamina; stem cells undergo rapid division (**stratum germinativum**) and gradually move towards surface (25-45 days)

Dermis - middle region **[B]**
- Strong, flexible connective tissue
- Cells include fibroblasts, macrophages, and occasionally mast cells and white blood cells

Papillary Layer [6]	• Areolar connective tissue with collagen and elastic fibers and blood vessels
	• **Dermal papillae** contain:
	  • Capillary loops
	  • Meissner's corpuscles
	• Free nerve endings

Reticular Layer [7]	• ~80% of the thickness of dermis • Collagen fibers provide strength and resiliency • **Elastic fibers provide stretch-recoil properties**

Hypodermis (superficial fascia) - deepest region **[C]**
- Subcutaneous layer deep to skin (not technically part of skin)
- Mostly adipose tissue

Figure 5.1 Layers of the skin

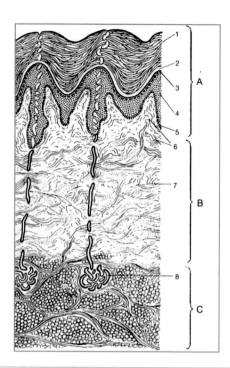

- **Friction Ridges** - Epidermal ridges lie atop deeper dermal papillary ridges to form friction ridges of **fingerprints**.
- **Cleavage Lines** - Collagen fibers arranged in bundles form cleavage (tension) lines
  - Incisions made parallel to cleavage lines heal more readily
- Three **pigments** contribute to **skin color**:
  - **Melanin**: Yellow to reddish-brown to black, responsible for dark skin colors
    - Produced in melanocytes; migrates to keratinocytes where it forms "pigment shields" for nuclei
  - **Freckles** and **pigmented moles**: Local accumulations of melanin
  - **Carotene**: Yellow to orange, most obvious in the palms and soles; taken in with food
  - **Hemoglobin**: Responsible for the pinkish hue of skin; in the blood, not the skin

Appendages of the skin

Sweat glands
- **Eccrine (merocrine) sweat glands** - abundant on palms, soles, and forehead; sweat (99% water, NaCl, vitamin C, antibodies, dermcidin, metabolic wastes) secreted via ducts **connected to pores**; function in **thermoregulation**
- **Apocrine sweat glands** - confined to axillary and anogenital areas; secrete **sebum** (sweat + fatty substances and proteins) via ducts **connected to hair follicles**; functional from puberty onward)
  - Specialized apocrine glands
    - **Ceruminous glands** - in external ear canal; secrete cerumen (deters insects)

- **Mammary (breast) glands**

Sebaceous (Oil) Glands
- Widely distributed
- Most develop from hair follicles
- Become active at puberty
  - **Sebum**: Oily holocrine secretion; bactericidal; softens hair and skin

Hair
- Consists of dead keratinized cells; **hard keratin** more durable than soft keratin of skin
- **Hair pigments**: melanins (yellow, rust brown, black)
  - **Gray/white hair**: decreased melanin production, increased air bubbles in shaft
- **Functions**: Alerting the body to presence of insects on the skin; guarding the scalp against physical trauma, heat loss, and sunlight
- **Distribution**: Entire surface except palms, soles, lips, nipples, and portions of external genitalia
- **Hair Follicle**: Extends from the epidermal surface into dermis
  - **Hair bulb**: expanded deep end
    - **Hair follicle receptor** (root hair plexus): Sensory nerve endings around each hair bulb
  - **Arrector pili**: Smooth muscle attached to follicle; responsible for "goose bumps"
- **Vellus hair** - pale, fine body hair of children and adult females
- **Terminal hair** - coarse, long hair of eyebrows, scalp, axillary, and pubic regions (and face and neck of males)

Nail – Scale-like modification of the epidermis on the distal, dorsal surface of fingers and toes

Functions of the Integumentary System

Protection - three types of barriers
- **Chemical**: Low pH secretions (acid mantle) and defensins retard bacterial activity
- **Physical/mechanical**: Keratin and glycolipids block most water and water-soluble substances; limited penetration of skin by lipid-soluble substances, plant oleoresins (e.g., poison ivy), organic solvents, salts of heavy metals, some drugs
- **Biological**: Dendritic cells, macrophages, and DNA

Body temperature regulation
- 500 ml/day of routine insensible perspiration (at normal body temperature)
- At elevated temperature, dilation of dermal vessels and increased sweat gland activity (sensible perspirations) cool the body

Cutaneous sensations - temperature, touch, and pain

Metabolic functions - Synthesis of vitamin D precursor and collagenase

Blood reservoir - up to 5% of body's blood volume

Excretion - nitrogenous wastes and salt in sweat

Skin Cancer

- **Most skin tumors are benign** (do not metastasize)
- **Risk factors**

- Overexposure to UV radiation
- Frequent irritation of the skin

Basal Cell Carcinoma
- Least malignant, most common
- Stratum basale cells proliferate and slowly invade dermis and hypodermis
- Cured by surgical excision in 99% of cases

Squamous Cell Carcinoma
- Second most common
- Involves keratinocytes of stratum spinosum
- Most common on scalp, ears, lower lip, and hands
- Good prognosis if treated by radiation therapy or removed surgically

Melanoma
- Most dangerous
- Involves melanocytes
- Highly metastatic and resistant to chemotherapy
- Treated by wide surgical excision accompanied by immunotherapy

Burn injuries

- Heat, electricity, radiation, certain chemicals (acid, lye) → tissue damage, denatured protein, cell death
- **Immediate threat**: Dehydration and electrolyte imbalance, leading to renal shutdown and circulatory shock
- After 48-72 hours threat from infection takes over

Partial-Thickness Burns
- **First degree** - Epidermal damage only
  - Localized redness, edema (swelling), and pain
  - Heals without problem
- **Second degree** - Epidermal and upper dermal damage
  - Blisters appear
  - Heals without problem as long as no infection of dermis

Full-Thickness Burns
- **Third degree** - Entire thickness of skin damaged
  - Gray-white, cherry red, or black
  - No initial edema or pain (nerve endings destroyed)
  - Skin grafting usually necessary

Rule of Nines - Used to estimate the extend of burn injury and volume of fluid loss
- The body surface is subdivided into 11 areas of 9% each
  - The head counts as one area of 9%
  - Each upper limb (arm) counts for 9% and each lower limb (leg) is counted as 18% (9% for the front of the leg and 9% for the back)
  - The front and back of the trunk count for 18% each, giving the trunk a total of 36%. The area over the front of the chest counts for 9% as does the area over the abdomen. On the back, the upper and lower back count for 9% each
  - The anogenital area makes up the remaining 1%

A&P Essentials 4th ed.

Chapter 6 Bones & Skeletal Tissues

Skeletal Cartilages

- Only dense connective tissue girdle of **perichondrium** contains blood vessels for nutrient delivery to cartilage
- **Hyaline cartilages**: Provide support, flexibility, and resilience; most abundant type
- **Elastic cartilages**: Similar to hyaline cartilages, but contain elastic fibers
- **Fibrocartilages**: Collagen fibers give great tensile strength
- **Appositional growth**: Cells secrete matrix against the external face of existing cartilage
- **Interstitial growth**: Chondrocytes divide and secrete new matrix, expanding cartilage from within

Calcification of cartilage occurs during normal bone growth and in **old age**

Bones

Classification by shape
- **Long bones**: Longer than they are wide
- **Short bones**: Cube-shaped bones (in wrist and ankle)
  - **Sesamoid bones** (within tendons, e.g., patella)
- **Flat bones**: Thin, flat, slightly curved
- **Irregular bones**: Complicated shapes

Functions of Bones
- **Support**: For the body and soft organs
- **Protection**: For brain, spinal cord, and vital organs
- **Movement**: Levers for muscle action
- **Storage**: Minerals (calcium and phosphorus) and growth factors
- **Blood cell formation** (hemopoiesis) in marrow cavities
- **Triglyceride (energy) storage** in bone cavities

Bone Textures
- **Compact bone**: Dense outer layer
- **Spongy (cancellous) bone**: Honeycomb of trabeculae

Structure of a Long Bone (see figure 6.1)
- **Diaphysis** (shaft): Compact bone collar surrounds **medullary (marrow) cavity**, which in adults contains fat (**yellow marrow**)
- **Epiphyses**: Expanded ends; spongy bone interior
  - **Epiphyseal line** (remnant of growth plate)
  - **Articular** (hyaline) **cartilage** on joint surfaces

Membranes of bone
- **Periosteum**
  - **Outer fibrous layer**
  - **Inner osteogenic layer**: Osteogenic (stem) cells, osteoblasts, osteoclasts
  - Nerve fibers, nutrient blood vessels, and lymphatic vessels enter the bone via nutrient foramina
  - Secured to underlying bone by **Sharpey's fibers**

- **Endosteum**: Delicate membrane on internal surfaces of bone
  - Also contains osteoblasts and osteoclasts

Structure of Short, Irregular, and Flat Bones
- Periosteum-covered **compact bone** on the outside
- Endosteum-covered **spongy bone** within
  - Spongy bone called **diploë** in flat bones
  - Bone marrow between the trabeculae

Figure 6.1 Long bone structure

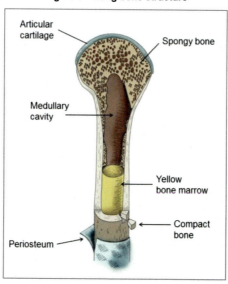

Bone Markings

Projections	
Projections that help to form joints	
Head	bony expansion carried on a narrow neck, e.g., neck of femur
Facet	smooth, nearly flat articular surface, e.g., facet of vertebra
Ramus	arm-like bar, e.g., pubic ramus
Condyle	Large, rounded articular projection, e.g., femoral condyles
Sites of muscle and ligament attachment	
Tuberosity	rounded projection, e.g., tibial tuberosity
Crest	narrow, prominent ridge, e.g., iliac crest
Trochanter	large, blunt, irregular surface, e.g., greater trochanter
Line (Linea)	narrow ridge of bone, e.g., linea aspera
Tubercle	small rounded projection, e.g., tubercle of humerus
Epicondyle	raised area above a condyle, e.g., medial femoral epicondyle
Spine	sharp, slender projection, e.g., anterior superior iliac spine
Process	any bony prominence, e.g., styloid process of ulna

A&P Essentials 4th ed.

Depressions and Openings	
Meatus	canal-like passageway, e.g., external acoustic meatus
Sinus	cavity within a bone, e.g., frontal sinus
Fossa	shallow, basin-like depression, e.g., mandibular fossa
Fissure	narrow, slit-like opening, e.g., sphenoid fissure
Foramen	round or oval opening through a bone, e.g., infraorbital foramen

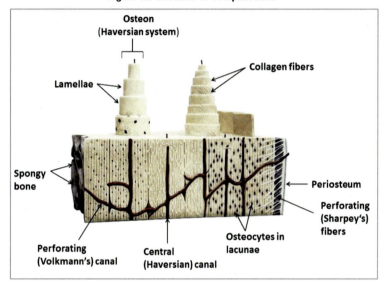

Figure 6.2 Structure of compact bone

Microscopic Anatomy

Cells of bones
- **Osteogenic (osteoprogenitor) cells**: Stem cells in periosteum and endosteum that give rise to osteoblasts
- **Osteoblasts**: Bone-forming cells
- **Osteocytes**: Mature bone cells
- **Osteoclasts**: Cells that break down (resorb) bone matrix

Compact Bone (see figure 6.2)
- **Haversian system** or **osteon** - structural unit
  - **Lamellae**: Weight-bearing, column-like matrix tubes
  - **Central (Haversian) canal**: Contains blood vessels and nerves
- **Perforating (Volkmann's) canals**: At right angles to the central canal; connect blood vessels and nerves of the periosteum and central canal
- **Lacunae** - small cavities that contain osteocytes
- **Canaliculi** – hair-like canals that connect lacunae to each other and the central canal

Spongy Bone
- **Trabeculae**: Align along lines of stress
  - No osteons

- Contain irregularly arranged lamellae, osteocytes, and canaliculi
- Capillaries in endosteum supply nutrients

Chemical Composition
- **Organic**
  - Osteogenic cells, osteoblasts, osteocytes, osteoclasts
  - **Osteoid** - organic bone matrix secreted by osteoblasts
    - **Ground substance** (proteoglycans, glycoproteins)
    - **Collagen fibers**: Provide tensile strength and flexibility
- **Inorganic**
  - **Hydroxyapatites** (mineral salts) - 65% of bone by mass
  - Mainly calcium phosphate crystals
  - Responsible for hardness and resistance to compression

Bone Development/Growth

Osteogenesis (ossification) - bone tissue formation
- **Bone formation** - begins in the 2nd month of development
- **Postnatal bone growth** - until early adulthood
- **Bone remodeling and repair** - lifelong

Two Types of Ossification
- **Intramembranous ossification**: Membrane bone develops from fibrous membrane
  - Forms flat bones, e.g. clavicles and cranial bones
- **Endochondral ossification**: Cartilage (endochondral) bone forms by replacing hyaline cartilage
  - Forms most of the rest of the skeleton
  - Uses hyaline cartilage models
  - Requires breakdown of hyaline cartilage prior to ossification

Postnatal Bone Growth
- **Interstitial growth**: ↑ length of long bones
- **Appositional growth**: ↑ thickness and remodeling of all bones by osteoblasts and osteoclasts on bone surfaces

Longitudinal Bone Growth
- Epiphyseal plate cartilage organizes into four important **functional zones**:
  - Proliferation (growth)
  - Hypertrophic
  - Calcification
  - Ossification (osteogenic)

Hormonal Regulation of Bone Growth
- **Growth hormone** stimulates epiphyseal plate activity
- **Thyroid hormone** modulates activity of growth hormone
- **Testosterone and estrogens** (at puberty) promote adolescent growth spurts; end growth by inducing epiphyseal plate closure

Bone Remodeling

Control of Remodeling

- Hormonal mechanisms that maintain calcium homeostasis in the blood
- Mechanical and gravitational forces

Hormonal Control of Blood Ca^{2+}
- Primarily controlled by **parathyroid hormone** (PTH):
  - ↓ Blood Ca^{2+} levels → **Parathyroid glands** release **PTH** → PTH stimulates **osteoclasts** to degrade bone matrix and release Ca^{2+} → ↑Blood Ca^{2+} levels
- May be affected to a lesser extent by **calcitonin**
  - ↑ Blood Ca^{2+} levels → **Parafollicular cells of thyroid** release **calcitonin** → **osteoblasts** deposit calcium salts → ↓Blood Ca^{2+} levels

Response to Mechanical Stress
- **Wolff's law**: A bone grows or remodels in response to forces or demands placed upon it → **Handedness** (right or left handed) results in bone of one upper limb being thicker and stronger; curved bones are thickest where they are most likely to buckle; large, bony projections occur where heavy, active muscles attach

Bone Fractures

Can be classified by four "either/or" classifications:
- Position of bone ends after fracture:
  - **Nondisplaced** - ends retain normal position
  - **Displaced** - ends out of normal alignment
- Completeness of the break
  - **Complete** - broken all the way through
  - **Incomplete** - not broken all the way through
- Orientation of the break to the long axis of the bone:
  - **Linear** - parallel to long axis of the bone
  - **Transverse** - perpendicular to long axis of the bone
- Whether or not the bone ends penetrate the skin:
  - **Compound** (open) - bone ends penetrate the skin
  - **Simple** (closed) - bone ends do not penetrate the skin

Stages of fracture healing
- **Hematoma**: Torn blood vessels hemorrhage → clot (hematoma) forms → site becomes swollen, painful, and inflamed
- **Fibrocartilaginous callus**: Phagocytic cells clear debris; osteoblasts begin forming spongy bone within 1 week; fibroblasts secrete collagen fibers to connect bone ends; mass of repair tissue now called fibrocartilaginous callus
- **Bony callus**: New trabeculae form a bony (hard) callus; continues until firm union is formed in ~2 months
- **Bone remodeling**: In response to mechanical stressors over several months; final structure resembles original

Homeostatic Imbalances of Bone Structure

Osteomalacia and rickets
- Calcium salts not deposited
- **Rickets** (childhood disease) causes bowed legs and other bone deformities

- **Cause**: vitamin D deficiency or insufficient dietary calcium

Osteoporosis
- Loss of bone mass - bone resorption outpaces deposit
- Spongy bone of spine and neck of femur become most susceptible to fracture
- **Risk factors**
  - Lack of estrogen, calcium or vitamin D
  - Petite body form
  - Immobility
  - Low levels of TSH
  - Diabetes mellitus
- **Treatment and Prevention**
  - Calcium, vitamin D, and fluoride supplements
  - ↑ Weight-bearing exercise throughout life
  - Hormone (estrogen) replacement therapy (HRT) slows bone loss
  - Some drugs increase bone mineral density

A&P Essentials 4th ed.

Chapter 7 Skeleton

Figure 7.1 Human Skeleton from the front (left) and back (right)

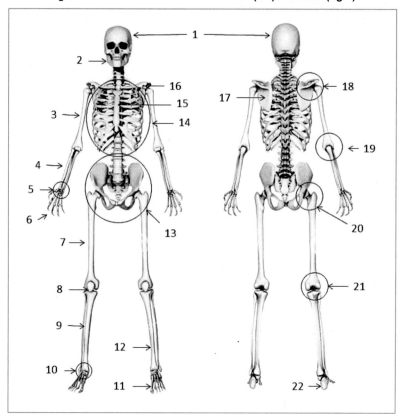

1. Skull
2. Mandible (jaw bone)
3. Humerus
4. Radius and ulna
5. Wrist with carpal bones
6. Digits with phalanges
7. Femur (thigh bone)
8. Patella (kneecap)
9. Fibula (calf bone)
10. Ankle with tarsal bones
11. Metatarsal bone
12. Tibia (shinbone)
13. Pelvis
14. Thoracic or rib cage
15. Sternum (breastbone)
16. Clavicle (collar bone)
17. Scapula (shoulder blade)
18. Shoulder
19. Elbow
20. Hip
21. Knee
22. Calcaneus (heel bone)

Bones of the Axial Skeleton

- **Skull – 22 bones**
  - **14 Facial bones**: Maxilla (2), palatine bone (2), zygomatic bone (2), lacrimal bone (2), nasal bone (2), vomer, inferior nasal concha (2), mandible

37

A&P Essentials 4th ed.

- **8 Cranial bones**: Frontal bone, parietal bone (2), occipital bone, temporal bone (2), sphenoid bone, ethmoid bone
- **Rib (thoracic) cage – 25 bones**: Ribs (24), sternum
- **Vertebral column – 26 bones**: Cervical vertebrae (7), thoracic vertebrae (12), lumbar vertebrae (5), sacrum, coccyx
- **Auditory ossicles – 6 bones**: Malleus (2), incus (2), stapes (2)
- **Hyoid – 1 bone**: Hyoid

Figure 7.2 Skull, anterior view

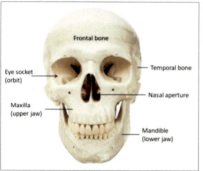

Figure 7.3 Skull, lateral view

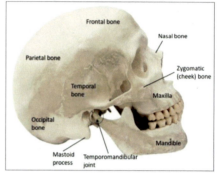

The Skull

8 Cranial bones: Enclose the brain in the **cranial cavity**
- **Cranial vault** (calvaria)
- **Cranial base**: anterior, middle, and posterior cranial fossae
- Provide sites of attachment for head and neck muscles

Frontal bone	• Anterior portion of cranium • Most of anterior cranial fossa • Superior wall of orbits • Contains air-filled frontal sinus

Parietal bones and associated sutures	• Superior and lateral aspects of cranial vault
	• Four sutures mark the articulations of parietal bones with frontal, occipital, and temporal bones:
	  • **Coronal suture** - between parietal bones and frontal bone
	  • **Sagittal suture** - between right and left parietal bones
	  • **Lambdoid suture** - between parietal bones and occipital bone
	  • **Squamous (squamosal) sutures** - between parietal and temporal bones on each side of skull

Occipital bone	• Most of skull's posterior wall and posterior cranial fossa • Surrounds **foramen magnum**

A&P Essentials 4th ed.

	• Articulates with 1st vertebra • Sites of attachment for the ligamentum nuchae and many neck and back muscles
Temporal bones	• Inferolateral aspects of skull and parts of cranial floor • Four major regions: Squamous, tympanic, mastoid with **mastoid process**, petrous

Sphenoid bone	• Complex, bat-shaped bone; articulates with all other cranial bones
	• Three pairs of processes
	  • **Greater wings**
	  • **Lesser wings**
	  • **Pterygoid processes**

Ethmoid bone	• Deepest skull bone • Superior part of nasal septum, roof of nasal cavities with cribriform plate for olfactory fibers • Contributes to medial wall of orbits

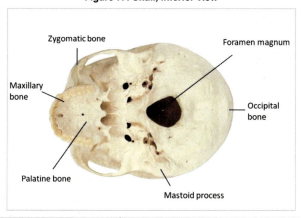

Figure 7.4 Skull, inferior view

14 Facial bones: Framework of face
• Cavities for special sense organs for sight, taste, and smell
• Openings for air and food passage
• Sites of attachment for teeth and muscles of facial expression

Mandible	• Lower jaw • Largest, strongest bone of face • **Temporomandibular joint**: only freely movable joint in skull
Maxillary bones	• Medially fused to form upper jaw and central portion of facial skeleton • Keystone bones: Articulate with all other facial bones except mandible
Zygomatic bones	• Cheekbones

Nasal bones	• Inferolateral margins of orbits • Form bridge of nose
Lacrimal bones	• In medial walls of orbits • Lacrimal fossa houses lacrimal sac
Palatine bones	• Posterior one-third of hard palate • Posterolateral walls of the nasal cavity • Small part of the orbits
Vomer	• Plow-shaped lower part of nasal septum
Inferior Nasal Conchae	• Form part of lateral walls of nasal cavity

Orbit

- Encases eyes and lacrimal glands
- Site of attachment for eye muscles
- Formed by parts of **seven bones**

Cranial bones
- Frontal bone
- Ethmoid bone
- Sphenoid bone

Facial bones
- Maxilla
- Lacrimal bone
- Zygomatic bone
- Palatine bone

Nasal Cavity

- **Roof, lateral walls, and floor** formed by parts of four bones
  - Ethmoid
  - Palatine bones
  - Maxillary bones
  - Inferior nasal conchae
- **Nasal septum** of bone and hyaline cartilage
  - Ethmoid
  - Vomer
  - Anterior septal cartilage

Paranasal Sinuses

- Mucosa-lined, air-filled spaces
- Lighten the skull
- Enhance resonance of voice
- Found in frontal, sphenoid, ethmoid, and maxillary bones

Hyoid Bone

- Does not articulate directly with another bone
- Site of attachment for muscles of swallowing and speech (suprahyoid and infrahyoid muscles)

Vertebral Column (numbers refer to figure 7.5)

- Transmits weight of trunk to lower limbs

- Surrounds and protects spinal cord

- Flexible curved structure containing **26 irregular bones** (vertebrae)
  - **Cervical vertebrae** (7) - vertebrae of the neck **[1]**
  - **Thoracic vertebrae** (12) - vertebrae of the thoracic cage **[2]**
  - **Lumbar vertebrae** (5) - vertebra of the lower back **[3]**
  - **Sacrum** - bone inferior to the lumbar vertebrae **[4]**
  - **Coccyx** - terminus of vertebral column **[5]**

- **Curvatures** increase the resilience and flexibility of the spine
  - Two posteriorly **concave curvatures**: Cervical and lumbar **[6, 7]**
  - Two posteriorly **convex curvatures**: Thoracic and sacral **[8, 9]**
  - **Abnormal spine curvatures**
    - **Scoliosis** (abnormal lateral curve)
    - **Kyphosis** (hunchback)
    - **Lordosis** (swayback)

Ligaments stabilize the spine
- **Anterior and posterior longitudinal ligaments**: From neck to sacrum
- **Ligamentum flavum**: Connects adjacent vertebrae; contains elastic fibers
- **Short ligaments**: Connect each vertebra to those above and below

Intervertebral Disc: Cushion-like pad composed of two parts
- **Nucleus pulposus**: Inner gelatinous nucleus that gives the disc its elasticity and compressibility
- **Anulus fibrosus**: Outer collar composed of collagen and fibrocartilage

Figure 7.5 Vertebral column (spine)

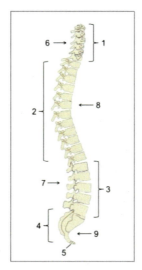

Vertebrae

General Structure of Vertebrae
- **Body or centrum**: Anterior weight-bearing region
- **Vertebral arch**: Composed of **pedicles** and **laminae** that, along with centrum, enclose vertebral foramen

- **Vertebral foramen**: Together make up **vertebral canal** for spinal cord
- **Intervertebral foramina**: Lateral openings between adjacent vertebrae for spinal nerves
- Seven processes per vertebra:
  - **Spinous process** - projects posteriorly
  - **Transverse processes** (2) - project laterally
  - **Superior articular processes** (2) - protrude superiorly inferiorly
  - **Inferior articular processes** (2) - protrude inferiorly

Figure 7.6 Vertebra (general structure)

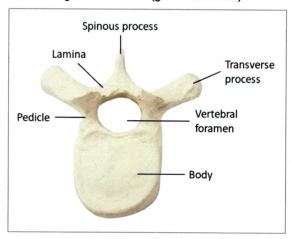

Cervical Vertebrae - C_1 to C_7: smallest, lightest vertebrae
- C_3 - C_7 share the following features
  - Oval body
  - Spinous processes are bifid (except C_7)
  - Large, triangular vertebral foramen
  - Transverse foramen in each transverse process
  - C_7 called **vertebra prominens** because of long spinous process; important landmark
- **Atlas (C_1)**
  - **No body** or spinous process
  - Consists of **anterior and posterior arches**, and two **lateral masses**
  - Superior surfaces of lateral masses articulate with the occipital condyles
- **Axis (C_2)**
  - **Dens** projects superiorly into the anterior arch of the atlas
  - Dens is a pivot for the rotation of the atlas

Thoracic Vertebrae - T_1 to T_{12}
- All articulate with ribs at facets and demifacets
- Long spinous process
- Location of articular facets allows rotation of this area of spine

Lumbar Vertebrae - L_1 to L_5

- Short, thick pedicles and laminae
- Flat hatchet-shaped spinous processes
- Orientation of articular facets locks lumbar vertebrae together to prevent rotation

Figure 7.7 Cervical vertebra, atlas and axis

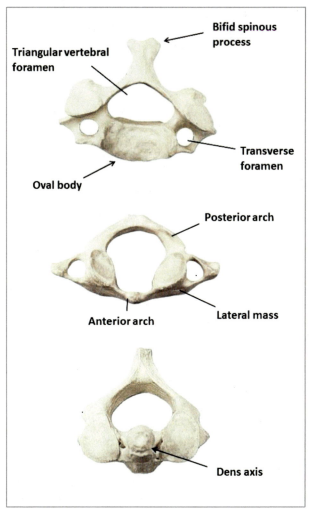

Sacrum and Coccyx

- **Sacrum**
  - 5 fused vertebrae (S_1–S_5)
  - Forms posterior wall of pelvis
  - Articulates with L_5 superiorly, and with auricular surfaces of the hip bones laterally
- **Coccyx** (Tailbone)
  - 3–5 fused vertebrae

- Articulates superiorly with sacrum

Figure 7.8 Thoracic cage

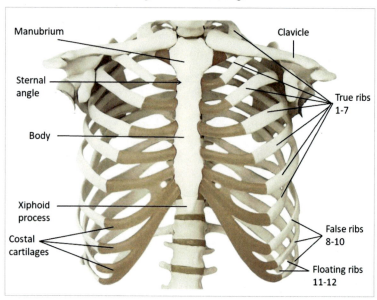

Thoracic cage

Functions   • Protects vital organs of thoracic cavity   • Supports shoulder girdle and upper limbs   • Provides attachment sites for many muscles, including intercostal muscles used during breathing
12 Thoracic vertebrae (see above)

Sternum (Breastbone)
 • Three fused bones
   • **Manubrium**: Articulates with clavicles and ribs 1 and 2
   • **Body**: Articulates with costal cartilages of ribs 2 through 7
   • **Stenal angle** between manubrium and body is important landmark; 2nd rib is to the left and right
   • **Xiphoid process**: Site of muscle attachment
     • Not ossified until ~ age 40

Ribs - 12 pairs   • All attach posteriorly to thoracic vertebrae   • **Pairs 1 through 7: True (vertebrosternal) ribs** - Attach directly to the sternum by individual costal cartilages   • **Pairs 8 through 12: False ribs**   • Pairs 8–10 also called **vertebrochondral ribs** - Attach indirectly to sternum by joining costal cartilage of rib above

- Pairs 11–12 also called **vertebral (floating) ribs**- No attachment to sternum

Structure of a Typical Rib
- **Head**: Articulates posteriorly with facets (demifacets) on bodies of two adjacent vertebrae
- **Neck**
- **Tubercle**: Articulates posteriorly with transverse costal facet of same-numbered thoracic vertebra
- **Shaft**

Bones of the Appendicular Skeleton

- **Pectoral girdle – 4 bones**: Scapula (2), clavicle (2)
- **Pelvic girdle – 2 bones**: Os coxae (2); each consisting of ilium, ischium and pubis
- **Upper extremity – 30 bones**: Humerus, radius, ulna, carpal bones (8): scaphoid, lunate, triquetrum, pisiform, trapezoid, trapezium, capitate and hamate, metacarpal bones (5), phalanges (14)
- **Lower extremity - 30 bones**: Femur, patella, tibia, fibula, tarsal bones (7): talus, calcaneus, navicular, cuboid, lateral, intermediate and medial cuneiform, metatarsal bones (5), phalanges (14)

Figure 7.9 Right shoulder girdle, anterior (left) and posterior (right) view

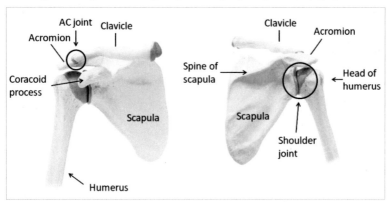

Pectoral (Shoulder) Girdle

- **Clavicles** and the **scapulae** attach the upper limbs to the axial skeleton
- Provide attachment sites for muscles that move the upper limbs

Clavicle (Collarbone)
- Flattened **acromial** (lateral) **end** articulates with the scapula
- Cone-shaped **sternal** (medial) **end** articulates with the sternum
- Acts as brace to hold the scapula and arm out laterally

Scapula (Shoulder Blade)
- Situated on the dorsal surface of rib cage, between ribs 2 and 7
- Flat and triangular, with three borders and three angles
- Seven large fossae, named according to location
- **Glenoid fossa** at the upper end of lateral border articulates with humerus to form

shoulder joint
- Above it is the beak-like **coracoid process**
- The **spine** on the posterior surface
- It ends in an enlarged process called **acromion**, which articulates with the lateral end of the clavicle

Upper Limb

- **30 bones** form the skeletal framework of each upper limb
  - **Arm** - Humerus
  - **Forearm** - Radius and ulna
  - **Hand** - 8 carpal bones in the wrist, 5 metacarpal bones in the palm, 14 phalanges in the fingers

Humerus

- Largest, longest bone of upper limb
- Proximal end forms a rounded, smooth **head** [1] that articulates superiorly with the glenoid cavity of scapula
- **Greater** [2] and **lesser tubercle** [3] and **deltoid tuberosity** [4] are attachment sites for muscles
- Distal end has **medial** and **lateral condyles** called **trochlea** [5] and **capitulum** [6] that articulate with radius and ulna
- **Medial** [7] and **lateral epicondyles** [8] are attachment sites for muscles
- Anterior aspect has two fossae, a shallow **radial** [9] and a deeper **coronoid fossa** [10]
- The **olecranon fossa** [11] is on the posterior aspect

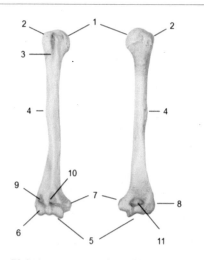

Right humerus, anterior (left) and posterior (right) view

Bones of the Forearm

Radius - Lateral bone in forearm
- The **head** articulates with capitulum of humerus and with radial notch of ulna
- **Radial tuberosity** is attachment site for biceps muscle
- Distal, expanded end is part of the wrist joint
- **Ulnar notch** on medial side articulates with ulna
- **Styloid process** on lateral side is anchoring side for ligaments
- Interosseous membrane connects the radius and ulna along their entire length

Ulna - Medial bone in forearm
- Forms the major portion of the elbow joint with the humerus
- **Olecranon** and **coronoid processes** at thick, proximal end separated by **trochlear notch**
- **Radial notch** articulates with head of radius
- Small distal end ends in lateral **head** and medial **styloid process**

A&P Essentials 4th ed.

Figure 7.10 Right forearm bones, anterior (left) and posterior (right) view

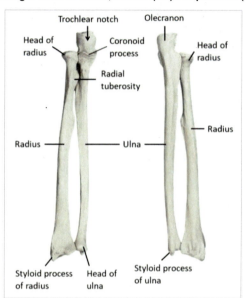

Bones of the Hand

Carpus - Eight bones in two rows
- **Proximal row** - Scaphoid, lunate, triquetrum, and pisiform
- **Distal row** - Trapezium, trapezoid, capitate, and hamate
  - Only scaphoid and lunate articulate with radius to form wrist joint

Metacarpus
- Five **metacarpal bones** (#1 to #5) form the palm

Phalanges – 14 bones
- Each **finger** (digit), except the thumb, has three phalanges - distal, middle, and proximal
- Fingers are numbered 1–5, beginning with the thumb
- **Thumb** (pollex) has no middle phalanx

Figure 7.11 Left hand, posterior view

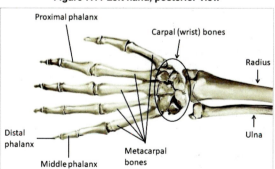

47

Pelvic (Hip) Girdle

- Two **hip bones** (also called **coxal bone** or os coxae) attach the lower limbs to the axial skeleton with strong ligaments
- Transmit weight of upper body to lower limbs
- Together with the **sacrum** and the **coccyx**, these bones form the **bony pelvis**

Hip Bone - Three regions
- **Ilium** - Superior region of the coxal bone
  - Upper wing-like **ala** ends in thickened **iliac crest**; medial surface forms **iliac fossa**
  - **Auricular surface** articulates with the sacrum (sacroiliac joint)
- **Ischium** - Posteroinferior part of hip bone
  - Two part: superior **body** and inferior **ramus** that connects with pubis and carries **ischial tuberosity**
- **Pubis** (pubic bone) - V-shaped anterior portion of hip bone with **inferior** and **superior ramus**
  - Bodies form **pubic symphysis** in the midline
- **Acetabulum**
  - Deep fossa were the bones fuse; articulates with the head of femur to form hip joint

Figure 7.12 Male pelvis, superior view

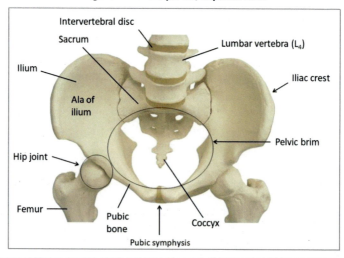

Pelvis
- True or lesser pelvis below the pelvic brim; defines birth canal
- False or greater pelvis above the brim

Comparison of Male and Female Pelvis

- **Female pelvis**
  - Adapted for childbearing
  - Cavity of the true pelvis is broad, shallow, and has greater capacity

- **Male pelvis**
  - Adapted for support of male's heavier build and stronger muscles
  - Cavity of true pelvis is narrow and deep
  - Tilted less forward

A&P Essentials 4th ed.

Lower Limb

- Carries the weight of the body
- **30 bones** form the skeletal framework of each lower limb
  - **Thigh** - femur
  - **Leg** - tibia and fibula
  - **Foot** - 7 tarsal bones, 5 metatarsal bones, 14 phalanges

Figure 7.13 Right femur, anterior (left) and posterior (right) view

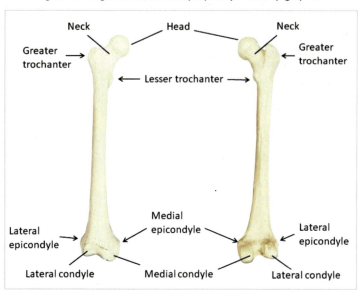

Femur and Patella

Femur - Largest and strongest bone in the body
- Articulates proximally with the acetabulum of the hip and distally with the tibia and patella
- Proximal end carries ball-like **head** on elongated neck; head articulates with acetabulum to form hip joint
- Lateral **greater trochanter** and posteromedial **lesser trochanter** are attachment sites for muscles
- Distal femur forms two wheel-like **medial and lateral condyles** each carrying a (medial and lateral) **epicondyle**
- The **patellar surface** is on the anterior aspect, the **intercondylar fossa** on the back

Patella (Kneecap) - Largest sesamoid bone of the body
- Triangular with the apex pointing down
- Embedded into the tendon of the quadriceps muscle
- **Patellar tendon** inserts into tibial tuberosity
- Cartilage-covered posterior surface part of femoropatellar joint

49

Bones of the Leg

Tibia (Shinbone)
- Triangular medial leg bone that receives the weight of the body from the femur and transmits it to the foot
- Broad, flat upper end subdivided by **intercondylar eminence** into **medial** and **lateral condyle**
- **Tibial tuberosity** attachment site for patellar ligament
- **Medial malleolus** forms bulge of the medial ankle
- **Fibular notch** articulates with fibula laterally

Fibula
- Not weight bearing; no articulation with femur
- Site of muscle attachment
- Connected to tibia by interosseous membrane
- Articulates with tibia via proximal and distal tibiofibular joints
- **Head** forms proximal end, **lateral malleolus** distal end and lateral ankle bulge

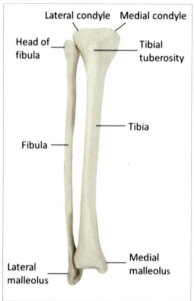

Figure 7.14 Right tibia and fibula, anterior view

Bones of the Foot

Tarsus
- Seven tarsal bones form the posterior half of the foot
- **Talus** (ankle bone) transfers most of the weight from the tibia to the calcaneus
- **Calcaneus** (heel bone), the biggest and strongest tarsal bone, is attachment site for Achilles tendon
- Other tarsal bones: **cuboid**, **navicular**, and the wedge-shaped **medial**, **intermediate**, and **lateral cuneiforms**

Metacarpus
- Five **metatarsal bones** (#1 to #5)
- Enlarged **head of metatarsal 1** forms the "ball of the foot"

Phalanges – 14 bones
- Each **toe** (digit), except hallux, has three phalanges - **distal**, **middle**, and **proximal**
- Toes are numbered 1–5, beginning with the hallux
- **Hallux** has no middle phalanx

Arches of the Foot
- Maintained by interlocking foot bones, ligaments, and tendons
- Allow the foot to bear weight
- **Three arches**
  - Lateral & medial longitudinal
  - Transverse

Figure 7.15 Left foot, superior view

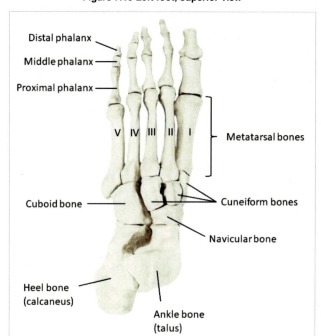

Chapter 8 Joints

Joint/Articulation - site where two bones or more meet

Functional Classification of Joints - Based on amount of movement allowed by the joint
- **Synarthroses** - immovable
- **Amphiarthroses** - slightly movable
- **Diarthroses** - freely movable

Structural Classification of Joints - Based on material binding bones together and whether or not a joint cavity is present
- **Fibrous Joints** - Bones joined by dense fibrous connective tissue; no joint cavity; most are synarthrotic (immovable)
  - **Sutures** - Rigid, interlocking joints containing short connective tissue fibers; allow for growth during youth; in middle age, sutures ossify and are called synostoses
  - **Syndesmoses** - Bones connected by ligaments (bands of fibrous tissue); movement varies from immovable to slightly movable
  - **Gomphoses** - Peg-in-socket joints of teeth in alveolar sockets; fibrous connection is the periodontal ligament
- **Cartilaginous Joints** - Bones united by cartilage; No joint cavity
  - **Synchondroses** - A bar or plate of hyaline cartilage unites the bones; all are synarthrotic
  - **Symphyses** - Hyaline cartilage covers the articulating surfaces and is fused to an intervening pad of fibrocartilage; strong, flexible amphiarthroses

Figure 8.1 Synovial joint

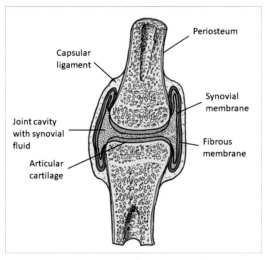

- **Synovial Joints**
  - Diarthrotic (freely movable); include all limb joints; most joints of the body
  - **Articular cartilage**: hyaline cartilage
  - **Joint (synovial) cavity**: small potential space

- **Articular (joint) capsule**: **Outer fibrous capsule** of dense irregular connective tissue and **Inner synovial membrane** of loose connective tissue
- **Synovial fluid** - Viscous slippery filtrate of plasma + hyaluronic acid; lubricates and nourishes articular cartilage
- **Three possible types of reinforcing ligaments:**
  - **Capsular** (intrinsic) - part of the fibrous capsule
  - **Extracapsular** - outside the capsule
  - **Intracapsular** - deep to capsule; covered by synovial membrane
- **Rich nerve and blood vessel supply:** Nerve fibers detect pain, monitor joint position and stretch; capillary beds produce filtrate for synovial fluid
- **Friction-Reducing Structures**
  - **Bursae:** Flattened, fibrous sacs lined with synovial membranes
    - Contain synovial fluid
    - Commonly act as "ball bearings" where ligaments, muscles, skin, tendons, or bones rub together
  - **Tendon sheath**: Elongated bursa that wraps completely around a tendon
- **Stabilizing Factors at Synovial Joints**
  - **Shapes of articular surfaces** (minor role)
  - **Ligament** number and location (limited role)
  - **Muscle tone**, which keeps tendons that cross the joint taut
    - Extremely important in reinforcing shoulder and knee joints and arches of the foot

Movements at Synovial Joints

Gliding Movements - One flat bone surface glides or slips over another similar surface

Angular Movements - Increase or decrease the angle between the articulating bones (joint angle)
- **Flexion** - decreases the angle of the joint
- **Extension** - increases the angle of the joint
- **Hyperextension** - excessive extension beyond normal range of motion
- **Abduction** - movement away from the midline
- **Adduction** - movement toward the midline
- **Dorsiflexion** - upward movement of the foot
- **Plantar flexion** - downward movement of the foot
- **Inversion** – turning the sole of the foot medially
- **Eversion** - turning the sole of the foot laterally
- **Protraction** - anterior movement of a body part in the horizontal plane
- **Retraction** - posterior movement of a body part in the horizontal plane
- **Elevation** - lifting a body part superiorly
- **Depression** - moving a body part inferiorly
- **Opposition** - movement in the saddle joint so that the thumb touches the tips of the other fingers

Circular Movements
- **Rotation** - turning of a bone around its own long axis
- **Pronation** - turning the hand forward

- **Supination** – turning the hand backward
- **Circumduction** - flexion + abduction + extension + adduction of a limb to describe a cone in space

Classification of Synovial Joints

- **Plane Joints** – nonaxial; flat articular surfaces; short gliding movements, e.ge., intercarpal joints
- **Hinge Joints** – uniaxial; motion along a single plane; flexion and extension only, e.g., elbow joint
- **Pivot Joints** – uniaxial; rounded end of one bone conforms to a "sleeve," or ring of another bone, e.g., atlantoaxial joint
- **Condyloid (Ellipsoidal) Joints** – biaxial; both articular surfaces are oval; permit all angular movements, e.g., wrist joint
- **Saddle Joints** – biaxial; each articular surface has both concave and convex areas; allow greater freedom of movement than condyloid joints, e.g., joint at the base of thumb
- **Ball-and-Socket Joints** – multiaxial; rounded convex surface of one bone articulates with cup-shaped surface of other bone; most freely movable joints, e.g., shoulder joint

Figure 8.2 Right shoulder joint, coronal section

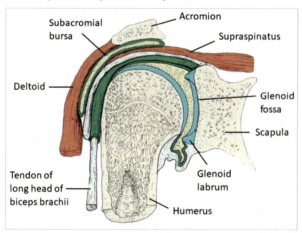

Shoulder Joint

- Ball-and-socket joint between **head of humerus** and **glenoid fossa** of the scapula
- **Glenoid labrum** increases contact surface
- **Reinforcing ligaments**:
    - **Coracohumeral ligament** - helps support the weight of the upper limb
    - Three **glenohumeral ligaments** - somewhat weak anterior reinforcements
- **Reinforcing muscle tendons**:
    - Tendon of the **long head of biceps** travels through the intertubercular groove
        - Secures the humerus to the glenoid cavity
- Four **rotator cuff** tendons encircle the shoulder joint: Supraspinatus, Infraspinatus, Teres minor, Subscapularis

Figure 8.3 Right elbow joint, sagittal section

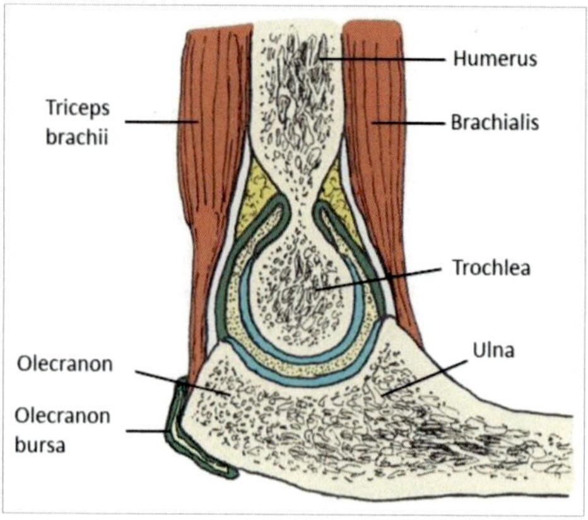

Elbow Joint

- **Hinge joint** formed mainly by trochlear notch of ulna and trochlea of humerus
- Flexion and extension only

- **Anular ligament** - surrounds head of radius
- Two capsular ligaments restrict side-to-side movement:
  - **Ulnar collateral ligament**
  - **Radial collateral ligament**

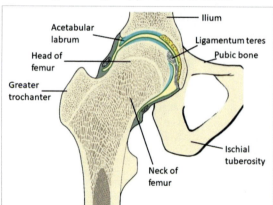

Figure 8.4 Right hip joint, coronal section

Hip (Coxal) Joint

- Ball-and-socket joint
  - **Head of the femur** articulates with the **acetabulum**
  - Good range of motion, but limited by the deep socket
  - **Acetabular labrum** - enhances depth of socket
- **Reinforcing ligaments**: Iliofemoral, pubofemoral, ischiofemoral ligament, ligamentum teres

Knee Joint

- Largest, most complex joint of body; three joints surrounded by a single joint cavity:
  - **Femoropatellar joint**: Plane joint; allows gliding motion during knee flexion
  - **Lateral and medial tibiofemoral joints** between the femoral condyles and the C-shaped **lateral and medial menisci** (semilunar cartilages) and the lateral and medial condyle of the tibia; allow flexion, extension, and some rotation when knee is partly flexed
- At least 12 associated **bursae**
- **Capsule** is reinforced by muscle tendons: e.g., quadriceps and semimembranosus tendons
  - **Joint capsule** is thin and absent anteriorly
  - Anteriorly, the quadriceps tendon gives rise to:
    - **Lateral and medial patellar retinacula**
    - **Patellar ligament** (inserts into tibial tuberosity)
- **Capsular and extracapsular ligaments**
  - Help prevent hyperextension
  - **Lateral (fibular) collateral ligament**
  - **Medial (tibial) collateral ligament** – fibers insert into medial meniscus
- **Intracapsular ligaments**:
  - **Anterior [ACL] and posterior cruciate ligaments [PCL]**
    - Prevent anterior-posterior displacement
    - Reside outside the synovial cavity

Figure 8.5 Right knee joint, anterior (left) and posterior (right) view

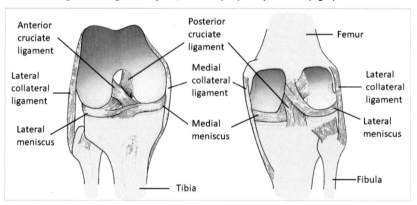

Temporomandibular Joint (TMJ)

- **Mandibular condyle** articulates with the **temporal bone**
  - **Hinge joint** - depression and elevation of mandible
  - **Gliding joint** - e.g. side-to-side (lateral excursion) grinding of teeth
- Most easily dislocated joint in the body due to of its unique structure and loose joint capsule

A&P Essentials 4th ed.

Chapter 9 Muscle Tissue

Special Characteristics of Muscle Tissue
- **Excitability** (responsiveness or irritability): ability to receive and respond to stimuli
- **Contractility**: ability to shorten when stimulated
- **Extensibility**: ability to be stretched
- **Elasticity**: ability to recoil to resting length

Three Types of Muscle Tissue

Skeletal muscle tissue:	Cardiac muscle tissue:	Smooth muscle tissue:
• Attached to bones and skin • Striated • Voluntary (i.e., conscious control) • Powerful	• Only in the heart • Striated • Involuntary • See Chapter 17 Heart Anatomy & Cardiac Muscle	• In the walls of hollow organs, e.g., stomach, urinary bladder, and airways • Not striated • Involuntary

Skeletal Muscles

- **Connective tissue sheaths** of skeletal muscle:
  - **Epimysium**: dense regular connective tissue surrounding entire muscle
  - **Perimysium**: fibrous connective tissue surrounding fascicles (groups of muscle fibers)
  - **Endomysium**: fine areolar connective tissue surrounding each muscle fiber
- Muscles attach:
  - **Directly** - epimysium of muscle is fused to the periosteum of bone or perichondrium of cartilage
  - **Indirectly** - connective tissue wrappings extend beyond the muscle as a ropelike **tendon** or sheetlike **aponeurosis**

Figure 9.1 Skeletal muscle cell/fiber

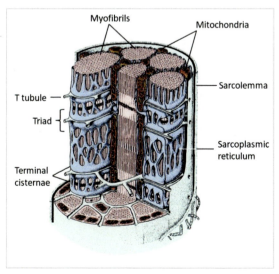

Microscopic Anatomy

- Cylindrical cell/fiber 10 to 100 μm in diameter, up to 12 inches (30 cm) long
- Multiple peripheral nuclei; many mitochondria
- Glycosomes for glycogen storage, myoglobin for O_2 storage

Myofibrils
- Densely packed, rodlike elements; ~80% of cell volume
- Exhibit **striations**: perfectly aligned repeating series of dark **A bands** and light **I bands**

Sarcomere
- The region of a myofibril between two successive Z discs; smallest contractile unit (functional unit) of a muscle fiber
- Composed of thick and thin myofilaments made of contractile proteins
- **Z disc**: coin-shaped sheet of proteins that anchors the thin filaments and connects myofibrils to one another
- **H zone**: lighter midregion where filaments do not overlap
- **M line**: line of protein myomesin that holds adjacent thick filaments together

Thick filaments run the entire length of an A band
- **Myosin tails** contain 2 interwoven, heavy polypeptide chains
- **Myosin heads** contain 2 smaller, light polypeptide chains that act as cross bridges during contraction
  - Binding sites for actin of thin filaments
  - Binding sites for ATP
  - ATPase enzymes

Thin filaments run the length of the I band and partway into the A band
- Twisted double strand of fibrous protein **F actin**
- F actin consists of **G** (globular) **actin** subunits
- G actin bears **active sites for myosin head** attachment during contraction
- **Tropomyosin** and **troponin**: regulatory proteins bound to actin

Sarcoplasmic Reticulum (SR)
- Network of smooth endoplasmic reticulum surrounding each myofibril
- Pairs of **terminal cisternae** form perpendicular cross channels
- Functions in the regulation of intracellular Ca^{2+} levels

T (transverse) Tubules - Continuous with the sarcolemma
- Penetrate the cell's interior at each A band–I band junction
- Associate with the paired terminal cisternae to form **triads** that encircle each sarcomere
  - T tubules conduct impulses deep into muscle fiber
  - Integral proteins protrude into the intermembrane space from T tubule and SR cisternae membranes
    - **T tubule proteins**: voltage sensors
    - **SR foot proteins**: gated channels; regulate Ca^{2+} release from SR cisternae

Figure 9.2 Myofibril

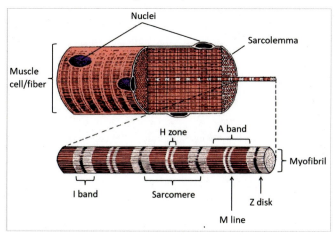

Figure 9.3 Sarcomere

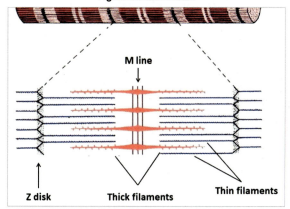

Contraction

Contraction = generation of force
- Does not necessarily cause shortening of the fiber! Shortening occurs when tension generated by cross bridges on the thin filaments exceeds forces opposing shortening

Neuromuscular Junction
- Skeletal muscles are stimulated by **somatic motor neurons**
- **Axons** of motor neurons travel from the central nervous system via **nerves** to skeletal muscles
- Each axon ending forms a **neuromuscular junction** with a single muscle fiber; axon and muscle fiber are separated by a gel-filled **synaptic cleft**
- **Synaptic vesicles** of axon terminal contain the neurotransmitter **acetylcholine** (ACh)
- Junctional folds of the sarcolemma contain **ACh receptors**
- Nerve impulse arrives at axon terminal → ACh is released and binds with receptors on the sarcolemma → electrical events lead to the generation of an **action potential**

- ACh effects are quickly terminated by the enzyme **acetylcholinesterase**

Requirements for Muscle Contraction
- **Activation**: neural stimulation at a **neuromuscular junction**
- **Generation and propagation of an action potential** along the sarcolemma
- **Final trigger**: a brief rise in intracellular Ca^{2+} levels

Generation of the Action Potential
- **Local depolarization (end plate potential):**
  - ACh binding opens chemically (ligand) gated ion channels → simultaneous diffusion of Na^+ (inward) and K^+ (outward)
  - More Na^+ diffuses, so the interior of the sarcolemma becomes less negative → **end plate potential**
- **Generation and propagation of an action potential:**
  - End plate potential spreads to adjacent membrane areas → voltage-gated Na^+ channels open → Na^+ influx decreases the membrane voltage toward a critical threshold → if threshold is reached, an **action potential** is generated
  - Local depolarization wave continues to spread, changing the permeability of the sarcolemma → voltage-regulated Na^+ channels open in the adjacent patch, causing it to depolarize to threshold
- **Repolarization:**
  - Na^+ channels close and voltage-gated K^+ channels open
  - K^+ efflux rapidly restores the resting polarity
  - Ionic conditions of the resting state are restored by the **Na^+-K^+ pump**

Sliding Filament Model of Contraction
- In the relaxed state, thin and thick filaments overlap only slightly
- During contraction, myosin heads bind to actin, detach, and bind again, to propel the thin filaments toward the M line
- As H zones shorten and disappear, sarcomeres shorten, muscle cells shorten, and the whole muscle shortens

Excitation-Contraction (E-C) Coupling
- Sequence of events by which transmission of an AP along the sarcolemma leads to sliding of the myofilaments
- AP is propagated along sarcomere to T tubules → voltage-sensitive proteins stimulate Ca^{2+} release from SR → Ca^{2+} binds to troponin → troponin changes shape and moves tropomyosin away from active sites → events of the **cross bridge cycle** occur
- When nervous stimulation ceases, Ca^{2+} is pumped back into the SR and contraction ends

Cross Bridge Cycle continues as long as Ca^{2+} and adequate ATP are present
- **Cross bridge formation** - high-energy myosin head attaches to thin filament
- **Working (power) stroke** - myosin head pivots and pulls thin filament toward M line
- **Cross bridge detachment** - ATP attaches to myosin head and the cross bridge detaches
- **"Cocking" of the myosin head** - energy from hydrolysis of ATP cocks the myosin head into the high-energy state

Muscle Mechanics

- Contraction produces tension, the force exerted on the load or object to be moved
- Contraction does not always shorten a muscle
- Force and duration of contraction vary in response to stimuli of different frequencies and intensities

Motor unit = a motor neuron and all (four to several hundred) muscle fibers it supplies
- **Small motor units** in muscles that control fine movements (fingers, eyes)
- **Large motor units** in large weight-bearing muscles (thighs, hips)
- Motor units in a muscle usually contract asynchronously; helps prevent fatigue

Muscle Twitch
- Response of a muscle to a single, brief threshold stimulus; simplest contraction observable in the lab
- Different strength and duration of twitches are due to variations in metabolic properties and enzymes between muscles
- Three phases of a twitch:
  - **Latent period**: events of excitation-contraction coupling
  - **Period of contraction**: cross bridge formation; tension increases
  - **Period of relaxation**: Ca^{2+} reentry into the SR; tension declines to zero

Graded Muscle Responses
- Variations in the degree of muscle contraction; required for proper control of skeletal movement
- Responses are graded by:
  - **Change in Stimulus Frequency**
    - Increased frequency of stimulus (muscle does not have time to completely relax between stimuli) → Ca^{2+} release stimulates further contraction → **temporal (wave) summation**
      - Further increase in stimulus frequency → **unfused (incomplete) tetanus**
      - If stimuli are given quickly enough, **fused (complete) tetanus** results
  - **Change in Stimulus Strength**
    - **Threshold stimulus**: stimulus strength at which the first observable muscle contraction occurs
    - Muscle contracts more vigorously as stimulus strength is increased above threshold
  - Contraction force is precisely controlled by **recruitment** (multiple motor unit summation), which brings more and more muscle fibers into action
  - **Size principle**: motor units with larger and larger fibers are recruited as stimulus intensity increases

Muscle Tone - Constant, slightly contracted state of all muscles; due to spinal reflexes that activate groups of motor units alternately in response to input from stretch receptors in muscles; keeps muscles firm, healthy, and ready to respond

Isometric Contractions: The load is greater than the tension the muscle is able to develop → tension increases to the muscle's capacity, but the **muscle neither shortens nor lengthens**

Isotonic Contractions: Muscle tension is greater than the load → **muscle changes in length and moves the load**

A&P Essentials 4th ed.

- **Concentric contractions** - the muscle shortens and does work
- **Eccentric contractions** - the muscle contracts as it lengthens

Muscle Metabolism

- ATP is the only source used directly for contractile activities
- Available **stores of ATP** are depleted in 4–6 seconds

Direct phosphorylation - Transfer of phosphate from creatine phosphate (CP) onto ADP → ATP

Anaerobic pathway (Glycolysis): Glucose → pyruvic acid + ATP
- At 70% of maximum contractile activity bulging muscles compress blood vessels → oxygen delivery is impaired → pyruvic acid is converted into lactic acid
- **Lactic acid**: Diffuses into the bloodstream; used as fuel by the liver, kidneys, and heart; converted back into pyruvic acid by the liver

Aerobic Pathway (Cellular respiration): Pyruvic acid → CO_2 + H_2O + ATP + Heat
- Produces 95% of ATP during rest and light to moderate exercise
- **Fuels**: stored glycogen, glucose, pyruvic acid, free fatty acids
- ~ 40% of the energy released in muscle activity is useful as work
- Remaining energy (60%) given off as heat
- Dangerous heat levels are prevented by radiation of heat from the skin and sweating

Oxygen Deficit = Extra O_2 needed after exercise for replenishment of
- Oxygen reserves
- Glycogen stores
- ATP and CP reserves
- Conversion of lactic acid to pyruvic acid, glucose, and glycogen

Muscle Fatigue - Physiological inability to contract
- Occurs when:
  - **Ionic imbalances** (K^+, Ca^{2+}, P_i) interfere with E-C coupling
  - Prolonged exercise damages the SR and interferes with Ca^{2+} regulation and release
  - **Total lack of ATP** occurs rarely during states of continuous contraction, and causes contractures (continuous contractions)

The **force of contraction** is affected by:
- Number of muscle fibers stimulated (**recruitment**)
- **Relative size of the fibers** - hypertrophy of cells increases strength
- **Frequency of stimulation** - ↑ frequency allows time for more effective transfer of tension to noncontractile components
- **Length-tension relationship** - muscles contract most strongly when muscle fibers are 80–120% of their normal resting length

Velocity and Duration of Contraction is influenced by:
- **Muscle Fiber Type** - Classified according to:
  - **Speed of contraction**: slow or fast, according to:
    - Speed at which myosin ATPases split ATP
    - Pattern of electrical activity of the motor neurons
  - **Metabolic pathways** for ATP synthesis:
    - **Oxidative fibers** - use aerobic pathways

- **Glycolytic fibers** - use anaerobic glycolysis
- **Slow oxidative fibers** – dark red (myoglobin), aerobic, fatigue-resistant, e.g., postural muscles
- **Fast oxidative fibers** – red–pink, aerobic, moderately fatigue-resistant, e.g., leg muscles
- **Fast glycolytic fibers** – white, anaerobic, fatigue fast, e.g., fibers in shoulder muscles
- **Load**: ↑ load → ↑ latent period, ↓ contraction, and ↓ duration of contraction
- **Recruitment**: → faster contraction and ↑ duration of contraction

Effects of exercise

Aerobic (endurance) exercise leads to increased:
- Muscle capillaries
- Number of mitochondria
- Myoglobin synthesis
- Results in greater endurance, strength, and resistance to fatigue
- May convert fast glycolytic fibers into fast oxidative fibers

Resistance exercise (typically anaerobic) results in:
- **Muscle hypertrophy** (due to increase in fiber size)
  - Increased mitochondria, myofilaments, glycogen stores, and connective tissue
  - **The Overload Principle**: Forcing a muscle to work hard promotes increased muscle strength and endurance → muscles adapt to increased demands
  - Muscles must be overloaded to produce further gains

Smooth muscle

- Found in walls of most hollow organs (except heart); usually in **two layers** (**longitudinal** and **circular**)
  - **Longitudinal layer** contracts; organ dilates and shortens
  - **Circular layer** contracts; organ constricts and elongates
- **Peristalsis**: Alternating contractions and relaxations of smooth muscle layers that mix and squeeze substances through the lumen of hollow organs

Microscopic Structure
- Thin, short, spindle-shaped fibers; endomysium only
- **SR**: less developed than in skeletal muscle; pouch-like infoldings (**caveolae**) of sarcolemma sequester Ca^{2+}; no sarcomeres, myofibrils, or T tubules
- **Myofilaments**
  - Ratio of thick to thin filaments (1:13) is much lower than in skeletal muscle (1:2)
  - Thick filaments have heads along their entire length
  - No troponin; protein **calmodulin** binds Ca^{2+}
  - Myofilaments are spirally arranged, causing smooth muscle to contract in a corkscrew manner
- **Dense bodies**: proteins that anchor noncontractile intermediate filaments to sarcolemma at regular intervals

Innervation of Smooth Muscle
- Autonomic nerve fibers innervate smooth muscle at diffuse junctions

- **Varicosities** (bulbous swellings) of nerve fibers store and release neurotransmitters

Contraction
- Slow, synchronized contractions; very energy efficient (slow ATPases)
- Cells are electrically coupled by **gap junctions**
  - Some cells are **self-excitatory** (depolarize without external stimuli); act as pacemakers for sheets of muscle; rate and intensity of contraction may be modified by neural and chemical stimuli
- **Sliding filament mechanism**; final trigger is ↑ intracellular Ca^{2+}; Ca^{2+} is obtained from the SR and extracellular space → Ca^{2+} binds to and activates calmodulin → activated calmodulin activates myosin (light chain) kinase → activated kinase phosphorylates and activates myosin
  - Cross bridges interact with actin
  - Myofilaments may maintain a **latch state** for prolonged contractions
- **Relaxation** requires Ca^{2+} detachment from calmodulin
  - Active transport of Ca^{2+} into SR and ECF
  - Dephosphorylation of myosin to reduce myosin ATPase activity

Regulation of Contraction
- **Neural regulation**: Neurotransmitter binding → ↑ $[Ca^{2+}]$ in sarcoplasm; either graded (local) potential or action potential
  - Response depends on neurotransmitter released and type of receptor molecules
- **Hormones and local chemicals**: May either enhance or inhibit Ca^{2+} entry

Special Features of Smooth Muscle Contraction
- **Stress-relaxation response**: Responds to stretch only briefly, then adapts to new length
  - Retains ability to contract on demand
  - Enables organs such as the stomach and bladder to temporarily store contents
- **Length and tension changes:** Can contract when between half and twice its resting length
- **Hyperplasia:** Smooth muscle cells can divide and increase their numbers, e.g., estrogen effects on uterus at puberty and during pregnancy

Types of Smooth muscle

- **Single-unit (visceral) smooth muscle**:
  - Sheets contract rhythmically as a unit (gap junctions)
  - Often exhibit spontaneous action potentials
  - Arranged in opposing sheets and exhibit stress-relaxation response

- **Multi-unit smooth muscle:**
  - Located in large airways, large arteries, arrector pili muscles, and iris of eye
  - Gap junctions are rare

Chapter 10 Muscular System

Functional Groups

- **Prime movers**: Provide the major force for producing a specific movement
- **Antagonists**: Oppose or reverse a particular movement
- **Synergists**: Add force to a movement; reduce undesirable or unnecessary movement
- **Fixators**: Synergists that immobilize a bone or muscle's origin

Lever Systems

Components of a lever system
- **Lever** - rigid bar (bone) that moves on a fixed point or fulcrum (joint)
- **Effort** - force (supplied by muscle contraction) applied to a lever to move a resistance (load)
- **Load** - resistance (bone + tissues + any added weight) moved by the effort

Classes of Lever Systems
- **First class**: Fulcrum between load and effort
- **Second class**: Load between fulcrum and effort
- **Third class**: Effort applied between fulcrum and load

Muscles of the Head

Muscles of Facial Expression: Insert into the skin; important in nonverbal communication; all innervated by cranial nerve VII **(facial nerve)**
- **Epicranius** (occipitofrontalis): Bipartite muscle consisting of the Frontalis and Occipitalis
  - **Galea aponeurotica** - cranial aponeurosis connecting them
  - The two muscles have alternate actions of pulling the scalp forward and backward

Muscles of Mastication and Tongue Movement
- **Prime movers of jaw closure**: Temporalis and masseter
- **Grinding movements**: Medial and lateral pterygoids
- All are innervated by cranial nerve V **(trigeminal nerve)**
- **Buccinator muscle** (of facial expression group) helps holding food between the teeth
- Three **muscles anchor and move the tongue**: Genioglossus, Hyoglossus, Styloglossus; all are innervated by cranial nerve XII **(hypoglossal nerve)**

Main muscles of facial expression and mastication

Muscle	Origin(s)	Insertion(s)	Action
Muscles of facial expression			
Frontalis	Galea aponeurotica	Skin of forehead/eyebrows	Wrinkles/elevates forehead and eyebrows
Orbicularis oculi	Bones of orbit	Tissue of eyelid, tarsal plate	Closes eyelid
Nasalis	Maxilla	Nasal cartilages	Flares nostrils
Orbicularis oris	Maxilla and mandible	Lips	Closes and purses lips
Levator labii superioris	Upper maxilla	Orbicularis oris and skin of upper lip	Elevates upper lip

A&P Essentials 4th ed.

Zygomaticus	Zygomatic bone	Superior corner of orbicularis oris	Elevates corner of mouth
Depressor labii inferioris	Mandible	Inferior corner of orbicularis oris	Depresses corner of mouth
Mentalis	Mandible	Skin of lower lip/chin	Depresses and protrudes lower lip
Buccinator	Maxilla and mandible	Orbicularis oris at angle of mouth	Compresses cheek to keep food between teeth
Muscles of mastication			
Temporalis	Temporal fossa	Coronoid process of mandible	Elevates mandible
Masseter	Zygomatic arch	Lateral ramus of mandible	Elevates mandible (prime mover)
Medial pterygoid	Sphenoid bone	Medial ramus of mandible	Elevates and laterally moves mandible
Lateral pterygoid	Sphenoid bone	Anterior side of condylar process of mandible	Protracts mandible
(Buccinator	Maxilla and mandible	Orbicularis oris at angle of mouth	Compresses cheek to keep food between teeth)

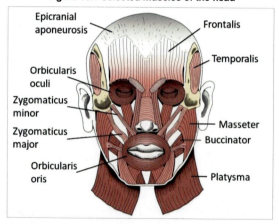

Figure 10.1 Selected muscles of the head

Muscles of the neck, throat and vertebral column

Muscles of the Anterior Neck and Throat: Most are involved in swallowing
• Two groups
• **Suprahyoid Muscles**
• **Infrahyoid Muscles**
Muscles of the Neck and Vertebral Column
• Two functional groups:
• **Muscles that move the head**
• **Muscles that extend the trunk and maintain posture**

Figure10.2 Muscles of the neck and throat, anterior view

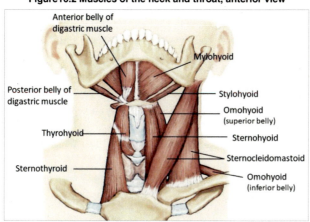

Muscles of the neck, throat and vertebral column

Muscle	Origin(s)	Insertion(s)	Action
Suprahyoid muscles - involved in swallowing (move hyoid bone and larynx)			
Digastric	Inferior border of mandible and mastoid process	Hyoid bone	Depresses mandible; elevates hyoid bone
Stylohyoid	Styloid process of temporal bone	Hyoid bone	Elevates and retracts hyoid
Mylohyoid	Inferior border of mandible	Hyoid bone	Elevates hyoid bone and floor of mouth
Geniohyoid	Medial surface of mandible at chin	Hyoid bone and median raphe	Elevates hyoid bone
Infrahyoid muscles - depress the hyoid and larynx			
Sternohyoid	Manubrium	Hyoid bone	Depresses hyoid bone
Sternothyroid	Manubrium	Thyroid cartilage	Depresses thyroid cartilage
Omohyoid	Superior border of scapula	Hyoid bone	Depresses hyoid bone
Thyrohyoid	Thyroid cartilage	Hyoid bone	Depresses hyoid bone; elevates thyroid cartilage
Muscles that move the head			
Sternocleidomastoid	Sternum and clavicle	Mastoid process	Flexes neck; rotates head to opposite side
Suprahyoid and infrahyoid muscles		Synergists to head flexion	
Scalene muscles		Lateral head movements	
Semispinalis capitis		Synergist with sternocleidomastoid	
Splenius (capitis and cervicis)		Head extension, rotation, and lateral bending	
Deep (intrinsic) back muscles			
Erector spinae (sacrospinalis) group		Prime movers of back extension and lateral	

[Iliocostalis, Longissimus, Spinalis]	bending
Semispinalis and **quadratus lumborum**	Synergists in extension and rotation

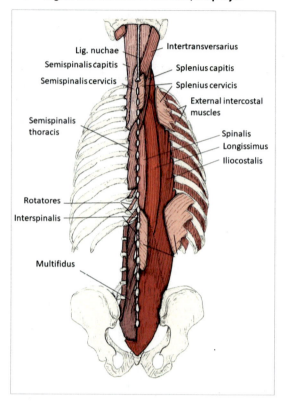

Figure 10.3 Muscles of the back, deep layer

Muscles of the Thorax

- **Muscles of respiration**
    - **External intercostals** - more superficial muscles that elevate ribs for inspiration
    - **Internal intercostals** - deeper muscles that aid forced expiration
    - **Diaphragm** - Partition between thoracic and abdominal cavities
        - Most important muscle in inspiration
        - Innervated by **phrenic nerve**

Muscles of the Abdominal Wall

- **Four paired muscles**, their fasciae and aponeuroses form the lateral and anterior abdominal wall
- Fascicles of these muscles run at angles to one another, providing added strength
- All are innervated by **intercostal nerves**
- **Actions** of these muscles
    - Lateral flexion and rotation of the trunk
- Help promote urination, defecation, childbirth, vomiting, coughing, and screaming

Muscle	Origin(s)	Insertion(s)	Action
External oblique	Lower eight ribs	Iliac crest and linea alba	Compresses abdomen; lateral rotation to opposite side
Internal oblique	Iliac crest, lumbodorsal fascia, inguinal ligament	Linea alba and costal cartilages of last 3-4 ribs	Compresses abdomen; lateral rotation
Transversus abdominis	Iliac crest, lumbodorsal fascia, costal cartilages of last 6 ribs	Xiphoid process, linea alba, pubic bone	Compresses abdomen
Rectus abdominis	Pubic crest and symphysis pubis	Xiphoid process, costal cartilages 5th-7th rib	Flexes vertebral column

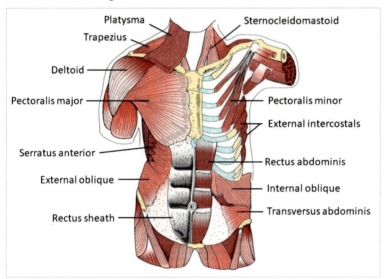

Figure 10.4 Muscles of the anterior trunk

Muscles of the pelvic wall and floor

- Pelvic floor (**pelvic diaphragm**) is composed of
  - **Levator ani**
  - **Coccygeus**
- Both are innervated by **sacral nerves**
  - Seals the inferior outlet of the pelvis
  - Supports pelvic organs
  - Lifts pelvic floor to help release feces
  - Resists increased intra-abdominal pressure
- **Muscles of the Perineum**
  - **Urogenital diaphragm**: Anterior half of perineum, inferior to pelvic floor
  - **Deep transverse perineal muscle**
  - **External urethral sphincter** (voluntary control of urination)

- **Muscles of superficial perineal space**: Ischiocavernosus, bulbospongiosus, superficial transverse perineal muscles, external anal sphincter (in posterior half of perineum)

Muscle	Origin(s)	Insertion(s)	Action
Obturator internus	Pelvic surface of ilium and ischium, obturator membrane	Greater trochanter	Rotates thigh laterally; assists in holding head of femur in acetabulum
Piriformis	Pelvis surface of S2-S4, superior margin of sciatic notch, sacrotuberous ligament	Greater trochanter	Rotates thigh laterally; abducts thigh; assists in holding head of femur in acetabulum
Levator ani (pubococcygeus, puborectalis, iliococcygeus)	Body of pubic bone, tendinous arch of obturator fascia, ischial spine	Coccyx, anococcygeal ligament, walls of prostate/vagina, rectum and anal canal	Forms most of pelvic diaphragm
Coccygeus	Ischial spine	Inferior end of sacrum and coccyx	Forms small part of pelvic diaphragm; flexes coccyx

Superficial Muscles of the Thorax

- Most are extrinsic shoulder muscles
- Act in combination to fix the shoulder girdle (mostly the scapula) and move it to increase range of arm movements
- Actions include elevation, depression, rotation, lateral and medial movements, protraction, and retraction
- **Two groups**: Anterior & posterior extrinsic shoulder muscles

Muscle	Origin(s)	Insertion(s)	Action
Anterior extrinsic shoulder muscles			
Pectoralis minor	Sternal end of ribs 3-5	Coracoid process of scapula	Pulls scapula forward and downward
Serratus anterior	Upper 8-9 ribs	Anterior medial border of scapula	Pulls scapula forward and upward
Subclavius	First rib	Subclavian groove of clavicle	Depresses clavicle
Pectoralis major	Clavicle, sternum costal cartilages 2-6	Greater tubercle of humerus	Flexes, adducts and rotates shoulder medially
Posterior extrinsic shoulder muscles			
Trapezius	Occipital bone and spines of cervical & thoracic vertebrae	Clavicle, acromion, and spine of scapula	Elevates, depresses and adducts scapula; hyperextends neck; braces shoulder
Levator scapulae	Cervical vertebrae 1-4	Superior border of scapula	Elevates scapula
Rhomboid major	Spines of thoracic vertebrae 2-5	Medial border of scapula	Elevates and adducts scapula

Rhomboid minor	Cervical (7th) and thoracic (1st) vertebrae	Medial border of scapula	Elevates and adducts scapula
Latissimus dorsi	Spines of sacral, lumbar and lower thoracic ribs, lower ribs	Intertubercular groove of humerus	Extends, adducts and laterally rotates humerus; adducts shoulder joint

Figure 10.5 Muscles of the posterior trunk

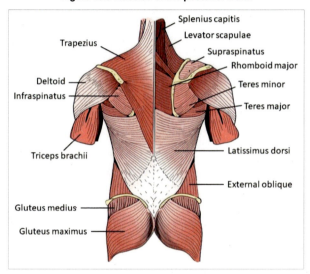

Muscles Crossing the Shoulder Joint

- Nine muscles cross the shoulder joint to insert on and move the humerus
- Some originate off the scapula; others originate off the axial skeleton
- Three are **prime movers of the arm**: Pectoralis major, latissimus dorsi, deltoid
  - Actions include flexion, extension, adduction, abduction, and rotation of humerus
- Four muscles are **rotator cuff muscles**: Supraspinatus, infraspinatus, teres minor, subscapularis
  - Reinforce the capsule of the shoulder
  - Act as synergists and fixators
- Two additional muscles are synergists: **coracobrachialis** and **teres major**

Muscle	Origin(s)	Insertion(s)	Action
Coracobrachialis	Coracoid process of scapula	Body of humerus	Flexes and adducts shoulder joint
Teres major	Inferior angle and lateral border of scapula	Intertubercular groove of humerus	Extends and rotates shoulder joint medially
Prime movers of the arm			
Pectoralis major	Clavicle, sternum costal cartilages 2-6	Greater tubercle of humerus	Flexes, adducts and rotates shoulder medially

Latissimus dorsi	Spines of sacral, lumbar and lower thoracic ribs, lower ribs	Intertubercular groove of humerus	Extends, adducts and laterally rotates humerus; adducts shoulder joint
Deltoid	Clavicle, acromion and spine of scapula	Deltoid tuberosity of humerus	Abducts, extends (anterior part) or flexes (posterior part) shoulder joint
Rotator cuff muscles			
Supraspinatus	Supraspinous fossa of scapula	Greater tubercle of humerus	Abducts shoulder joint
Infraspinatus	Infraspinous fossa of scapula	Greater tubercle of humerus	Rotates arm laterally; assists in keeping humeral head in glenoid cavity
Teres minor	Lateral border of scapula	Greater tubercle of humerus	Rotates arm laterally; assists in keeping humeral head in glenoid cavity
Subscapularis	Subscapular fossa	Lesser tubercle of humerus	Adducts and rotates arm medially; assists in keeping humeral head in glenoid cavity

Figure 10.6 Muscles of the upper limb, anterior and posterior view

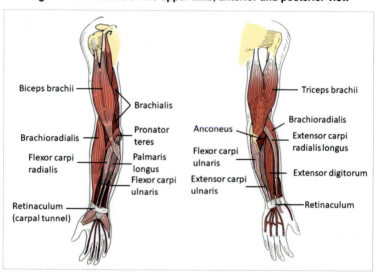

Muscles crossing the elbow joint

- **Anterior flexor muscles**
  - **Brachialis** and **biceps brachii** - chief forearm flexors
  - **Brachioradialis** - synergist and stabilizer
- **Posterior extensor muscles**
  - **Triceps brachii** - prime mover of forearm extension

- **Anconeus** - weak synergist

Muscle	Origin(s)	Insertion(s)	Action
Anterior flexor muscles			
Biceps brachii	Coracoid process and tuberosity above glenoid fossa	Radial tuberosity	Flexes elbow joint; supinates forearm and hand at radioulnar joint
Brachialis	Anterior body of humerus	Tuberosity of ulna	Flexes elbow joint
Brachioradialis	Lateral supracondylar ridge of humerus	Proximal to styloid process of radius	Flexes elbow joint
Posterior extensor muscles			
Triceps brachii	Tuberosity below glenoid fossa; lateral and medial surfaces of humerus	Olecranon of ulna	Extends elbow joint
Anconeus	Lateral epicondyle of humerus	Olecranon of ulna	Extends elbow joint

Muscles of the Forearm

- **Actions**: movements of the wrist, hand, and fingers
  - Most anterior muscles are flexors and insert via the **flexor retinaculum**
  - Most posterior muscles are extensors and insert via the **extensor retinaculum**
  - **Pronators**: pronator teres and pronator quadratus
  - **Supinator**: a synergist with the biceps brachii
  - **Anterior Compartment** – Flexors (innervated by median and ulnar nerve)
  - **Posterior Compartment** - Extensors (innervated by radial nerve)

Muscle	Origin(s)	Insertion(s)	Action
Supinator	Lateral epicondyle of humerus and crest of ulna	Lateral surface of radius	Supinates forearm and hand
Pronator teres	Medial epicondyle of humerus	Lateral surface of radius	Pronates forearm and hand
Pronator quadratus	Distal fourth of ulna	Distal fourth of radius	Pronates forearm and hand
Anterior compartment			
Flexor carpi radialis	Medial epicondyle of humerus	Base of metacarpal bone 2 and 3	Flexes and abducts wrist
Palmaris longus	Medial epicondyle of humerus	Palmar aponeurosis	Flexes wrist
Flexor carpi ulnaris	Medial epicondyle of humerus and olecranon of ulna	Carpal and metacarpal bones	Flexes and adducts wrist
Flexor digitorum superficialis	Medial epicondyle of humerus and coronoid process of ulna	Middle phalanges of digits 2-5	Flexes wrist and digits

Muscle	Origin(s)	Insertion(s)	Action
Flexor digitorum profundus	Proximal 2/3 of ulna and interosseous membrane	Distal phalanges of digits 2-5	Flexes wrist and digits
Flexor pollicis longus	Body of radius and coronoid process of ulna	Distal phalanx of thumb	Flexes thumb
Posterior Compartment			
Extensor carpi radialis longus	Lateral supracondylar ridge of humerus	2nd metacarpal bone	Extends and abducts wrist
Extensor carpi radialis brevis	Lateral epicondyle of humerus	3rd metacarpal bone	Extends and abducts wrist
Extensor digitorum	Lateral epicondyle of humerus	Posterior surfaces of digits 2-5	Extends wrist and phalanges
Extensor carpi ulnaris	Lateral epicondyle of humerus and olecranon of ulna	Base of 5th metacarpal bone	Extends and adducts wrist
Extensor pollicis brevis	Distal body of radius and interosseous membrane	Base of proximal phalanx of thumb	Extends thumb; abducts hand
Extensor pollicis longus	Lateral and posterior surface of ulna	Base of distal phalanx of thumb	Extends thumb; abducts hand
Extensor indicis	Posterior surface of ulna and interosseous membrane	2nd digit	Extends index
Abductor pollicis longus	Distal radius and ulna and interosseous membrane	Base of 1st metacarpal bone	Abducts thumb and hand

Intrinsic Muscles of the Hand

- Small weak muscles; lie entirely within the palm of the hand; control precise movements of metacarpals and fingers; abductors and adductors of the fingers; produce opposition - move the thumb toward the little finger
- **Thenar eminence** (ball of the thumb) and **hypothenar eminence** (ball of the little finger) have a flexor, an abductor, and an opponens muscle
- **Midpalmar muscles**: lumbricals and palmar and dorsal interossei extend the fingers
  - Interossei muscles also abduct and adduct the fingers

Muscles Crossing Hip and Knee Joints

- Most **anterior muscles flex the femur at the hip and extend the leg at the knee** (foreswing of walking)
- Most **posterior muscles extend the thigh and flex the leg** (backswing of walking)
- **Medial muscles adduct** the thigh
- All enclosed by **fascia lata**; thickens distally and forms flexor, extensor and fibular retinaculae

Muscle	Origin(s)	Insertion(s)	Action
Thigh flexors pass in front of the hip joint; assisted by medial adductors			

	Origin	Insertion	Function
Iliopsoas (iliacus and psoas major)	Iliac fossa (iliacus) and transverse processes of lumbar vertebrae (psoas major)	Lesser trochanter of femur	Prime mover of hip flexion; flexes joints of vertebral column
Tensor fasciae latae	Anterior border of ilium and iliac crest	Iliotibial tract	Abducts and rotates thigh medially
Rectus femoris	Anterior inferior iliac spine	Tibial tuberosity via patellar tendon	Flexes hip; extends leg at knee
Sartorius	Anterior superior iliac spine	Medial surface of tibia	Flexes leg and thigh; abducts and rotates thigh laterally
Thigh extensors			
Hamstrings (biceps femoris, semitendinosus, semimembranosus)	Ischial tuberosity and linea aspera of femur (short head of biceps)	Head of fibula and proximal lateral part of tibia (biceps) or proximal medial surface of tibia	Prime mover for extension of thigh at hip and flexion of leg at knee
Gluteus maximus	Iliac crest, sacrum, coccyx and aponeurosis of lumbar region	Gluteal tuberosity and iliotibial tract	Prime mover during forceful extension of thigh at hip; rotates thigh laterally
Adductors (also medially rotate thigh)			
Adductor magnus	Inferior rami of ischium and pubis	Linea aspera and medial epicondyle of femur	Adducts thigh at hip
Adductor longus	Pubis below pubic crest	Linea aspera	Adducts thigh at hip
Adductor brevis	Inferior ramus of pubis	Linea aspera	Adducts thigh at hip
Pectineus	Pectineal line of pubis	Distal to lesser trochanter of femur	Adducts and flexes thigh at hip
Gracilis	Inferior edge of symphysis pubis	Proximal medial surface of tibia	Adducts thigh at hip; flexes leg at knee
Abductors			
Gluteus maximus	Iliac crest, sacrum, coccyx and aponeurosis of lumbar region	Gluteal tuberosity and iliotibial tract	Prime mover during forceful extension of thigh at hip; rotates thigh laterally
Gluteus medius	Lateral surface of ilium	Greater trochanter	Abducts and medially rotates thigh
Gluteus minimus	Lateral surface of the lower half of ilium	Greater trochanter	Abducts and medially rotates thigh
Piriformis	Anterior surface of sacrum and sacrotuberous ligament	Femoral nerve	Rotates thigh laterally; abducts thigh; assists in holding head of femur in acetabulum
Obturator externus	Obturator foramen and membrane	Trochanteric fossa of femur	Rotates thigh laterally; abducts thigh; assists in holding head of femur in

			acetabulum
Obturator internus	Pelvic surface of obturator membrane	Greater trochanter	Rotates thigh laterally; abducts thigh; assists in holding head of femur in acetabulum
Gemellus superior and inferior	Ischial spine and tuberosity	Greater trochanter	Rotates thigh laterally; abducts thigh; assists in holding head of femur in acetabulum
Thigh muscles that move the knee joint			
Quadriceps femoris (rectus femoris, vastus lateralis, intermedius and medialis)	Anterior inferior iliac spine (rectus femoris), femur	Tibial tuberosity via patellar tendon	Prime mover for extension of the leg at knee joint
Hamstrings (biceps femoris, semitendinosus, semimembranosus)	Ischial tuberosity and linea aspera of femur (short head of biceps)	Head of fibula and proximal lateral part of tibia (biceps) or proximal medial surface of tibia	Prime mover for extension of thigh at hip joint and flexion of leg at knee joint

Figure 10.7 Muscles of the lower limb, anterior and posterior view

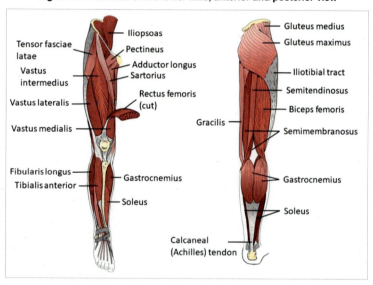

Muscles of the Leg and Foot

- Various leg muscles produce the following movements
  - **Ankle** - dorsiflexion and plantar flexion
  - **Intertarsal joints** - inversion and eversion of the foot
  - **Toes** - flexion and extension
- **Intrinsic Muscles of the Foot** - Help flex, extend, abduct, and adduct the toes; support the arches of the foot along with some leg tendons
  - **Extensor digitorum brevis** - dorsal foot muscle that helps extend the toes

Muscle	Origin(s)	Insertion(s)	Action
Anterior compartment - Primary toe extensors and ankle dorsiflexors			
Tibialis anterior	Lateral condyle and body of tibia	1st metatarsal and 1st cuneiform bone	Dorsiflexes ankle; inverts foot and ankle
Extensor digitorum longus	Lateral condyle of tibia and anterior surface of fibula	Middle and distal phalanges of digits 2-5	Extends digits 2-5; dorsiflexes ankle
Extensor hallucis longus	Anterior surface of fibula and interosseous membrane	Distal phalanx of hallux	Extends hallux; dorsiflexes ankle
Fibularis tertius (not always present)	Anterior surface of fibula and interosseous membrane	Dorsal surface of 5th metatarsal bone	Dorsiflexes ankle; everts foot and ankle
Lateral compartment - Plantar flexion and eversion of the foot			
Fibularis longus	Lateral condyle of tibia and head and shaft of fibula	Medial cuneiform and 1st metatarsal bone	Plantar flexes and everts foot
Fibularis brevis	Inferior 2/3 of fibula	5th metatarsal bone	Plantar flexes and everts foot
Posterior compartment - Flexors of the foot and the toes			
Gastrocnemius	Lateral and medial condyle of femur	Calcaneus via calcaneal tendon	Plantar flexes foot at ankle; raises heel during walking; flexes leg at knee joint
Soleus	Posterior aspect of fibula and tibia	Calcaneus via calcaneal tendon	Plantar flexes foot at ankle
Plantaris	Supracondylar ridge of femur	Calcaneus	Plantar flexes foot at ankle
Popliteus	Lateral condyle of femur	Upper posterior aspect of tibia	Flexes and medially rotates knee joint
Tibialis posterior	Tibia, fibula and interosseous membrane	Navicular, cuneiform, cuboid and metatarsal bones 2-4	Plantar flexes and inverts foot at ankle; supports arches of foot
Flexor digitorum longus	Posterior surface of tibia	Distal phalanges digits 2-5	Plantar flexes foot at ankle; flexes digits 2-5; supports longitudinal arches of foot
Flexor hallucis longus	Posterior surface of tibia	Distal phalanx of hallux	Plantar flexes foot at ankle; flexes hallux; supports medial longitudinal arch of foot

Chapter 11 Nervous Tissue

Functions of the Nervous System
- **Sensory input**: Information gathered by sensory receptors about internal and external changes
- **Integration**: Interpretation of sensory input
- **Motor output**: Activation of effector organs (muscles and glands) produces a response

Divisions of the Nervous System
- **Central nervous system** (CNS) - Brain and spinal cord
  - Integration and command center
- **Peripheral nervous system** (PNS): Paired **spinal and cranial nerves** carry messages to and from the CNS
  - Sensory (afferent) division
    - Somatic afferent fibers - convey impulses from skin, skeletal muscles, and joints
    - Visceral afferent fibers - convey impulses from visceral organs
  - Motor (efferent) division: Transmits impulses from the CNS to effector organs
    - Somatic (voluntary) nervous system: Conscious control of skeletal muscles
    - Autonomic (involuntary) nervous system (ANS)
      - Visceral motor nerve fibers regulate smooth muscle, cardiac muscle, and glands
      - Two functional subdivisions
        - Sympathetic
        - Parasympathetic

Figure 11.1 Overview over the nervous system

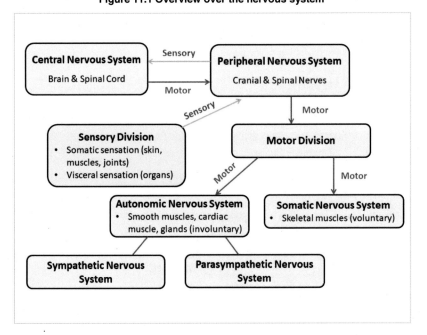

Histology of Nervous Tissue

Neuroglia (glial cells) - supporting cells
- **CNS**: Astrocytes, microglia, ependymal cells, oligodendrocytes
- **PNS**: satellite cells, Schwann cells

Astrocytes	• Most abundant, versatile, and highly branched glial cells • Cling to neurons, synaptic endings, and capillaries • Support and brace neurons • Help determine capillary permeability • Guide migration of young neurons • Control the chemical environment • Participate in information processing in the brain
Microglia	• Small, ovoid cells with thorny processes • Migrate toward injured neurons • Phagocytize microorganisms and neuronal debris
Ependymal Cells	• Line the central cavities of the brain and spinal column; May be ciliated • Separate the CNS interstitial fluid from the cerebrospinal fluid in the cavities
Oligodendrocytes	• Processes wrap CNS nerve fibers, form myelin sheaths
Satellite cells	• Surround neuron cell bodies in the PNS
Schwann cells (neurolemmocytes)	• Surround peripheral nerve fibers and form myelin sheaths • Vital to regeneration of damaged peripheral nerve fibers

Neurons (Nerve Cells)
- Excitable cells that transmit electrical signals
- **Special characteristics**:
  - Long-lived; amitotic - with few exceptions; high metabolic rate - depends on continuous supply of oxygen and glucose
  - Plasma membrane functions in:
    - Electrical signaling
    - Cell-to-cell interactions during development

- **Cell Body** (Perikaryon or Soma): Biosynthetic center of a neuron
  - Spherical nucleus with nucleolus; well-developed Golgi apparatus
  - Rough ER called **Nissl bodies** (chromatophilic substance)
  - Network of neurofibrils (neurofilaments)
  - **Axon hillock** - cone-shaped area from which axon arises

- **Processes**: Dendrites and axons
  - **Dendrites**: Short, tapering, and diffusely branched
    - Receptive (input) region of a neuron
    - Convey electrical signals toward the cell body as graded potentials
  - **Axon**: One axon per cell arising from the axon hillock
    - Long axons (nerve fibers); occasional branches (axon collaterals)
    - Numerous **terminal branches** (telodendria); knoblike **axon terminals** (synaptic knobs or boutons); secretory region of neuron, release **neurotransmitters** to ex-

cite or inhibit other cells
- Conducting region of a neuron; generates and transmits nerve impulses (action potentials) away from the cell body
- Molecules and organelles are moved along axons by motor molecules in two directions:
  - **Anterograde** - toward axonal terminal, e.g., mitochondria, membrane components, enzymes
  - **Retrograde** - toward the cell body, e.g., organelles to be degraded, signal molecules, viruses, and bacterial toxins

- **Myelin Sheath**: Segmented protein-lipoid sheath around most long or large-diameter axons; protects and electrically insulates the axon; increases speed of nerve impulse transmission
- **Myelin Sheaths in the PNS**: Schwann cells wraps many times around the axon
  - **Neurilemma** - peripheral bulge of Schwann cell cytoplasm
  - **Nodes of Ranvier**: Myelin sheath gaps between adjacent Schwann cells
    - Sites where axon collaterals can emerge
- **Myelin Sheaths in the CNS**: Formed by processes of oligodendrocytes; nodes of Ranvier are present

Unmyelinated Axons
- Thin nerve fibers are unmyelinated
- One Schwann cell may incompletely enclose 15 or more unmyelinated axons

- **Clusters of cell bodies** are called **nuclei** in the CNS and **ganglia** in the PNS
- **Bundles of processes** are called **tracts** in the CNS and **nerves** in the PNS
- **White matter**: Dense collections of myelinated fibers
- **Gray matter**: Mostly neuron cell bodies and unmyelinated fibers

Figure 11.2 Multipolar neuron with myelinated axon

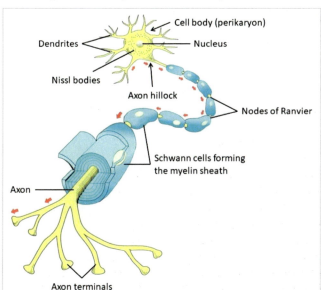

Structural Classification of Neurons
- **Multipolar** - 1 axon and several dendrites; most abundant; motor neurons and interneurons
- **Bipolar** - 1 axon and 1 dendrite; rare, e.g., retinal neurons
- **Unipolar (pseudounipolar)** - single, short process that has two branches:
  - **Peripheral process** - more distal branch, often associated with a sensory receptor
  - **Central process** - branch entering the CNS

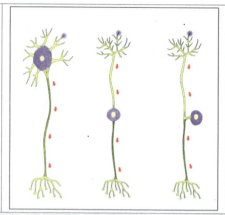

The **SAM** (or **ACE**) **classification** is **based on the function of neurons**:
- **Sensory (Afferent) neurons**: Transmit impulses from sensory receptors toward the CNS
- **Association (Connecting) neurons** link sensory and motor neurons. Association neurons are sometimes also referred to as **interneurons**
- **Motor (Efferent) neurons** carry impulses *away* from the CNS to muscles and glands

The conduction velocity of neurons varies widely
- Larger diameter fibers have less resistance to local current flow and have faster impulse conduction
- Conduction in unmyelinated axons is slower than **saltatory conduction** in myelinated axons
- saltatory conduction in myelinated axons is up to 100 times faster than signal conduction in non-myelinated fibers

Synapses

- A junction that mediates information transfer from one neuron to another neuron, or to an effector cell
  - **Presynaptic neuron** - conducts impulses toward the synapse
  - **Postsynaptic neuron** - transmits impulses away from the synapse

- Types of Synapses
  - **Axodendritic** - between axon and dendrite
  - **Axosomatic** - between axon and soma
  - **Axoaxonic** - axon to axon
  - **Dendrodendritic** - dendrite to dendrite
  - **Dendrosomatic** - dendrite to soma

Electrical Synapses - Neurons are electrically coupled (joined by gap junctions)
- Communication is very rapid, and may be unidirectional or bidirectional

Chemical Synapses - Specialized for the release and reception of neurotransmitters
- Typically composed of two parts
  - **Axon terminal** of the presynaptic neuron, which contains synaptic vesicles
  - **Receptor region** on the postsynaptic neuron

- **Synaptic Cleft** - Fluid-filled space separating the neurons
  - Prevents nerve impulses from directly passing from one neuron to the next
  - Transmission across the synaptic cleft is a chemical event involving release, diffusion, and binding of neurotransmitters
  - Ensures unidirectional communication between neurons
- **Information Transfer**
  - AP arrives at axon terminal of the presynaptic neuron and opens voltage-gated Ca^{2+} channels → promotes fusion of synaptic vesicles with axon membrane → exocytosis of neurotransmitter → diffuses and binds to receptors on the postsynaptic neuron → ion channels are opened, causing a graded potential)
- **Termination of Neurotransmitter Effects**
  - Degradation by enzymes
  - Reuptake by astrocytes or axon terminal
  - Diffusion away from the synaptic cleft
- **Synaptic Delay**
  - Neurotransmitter must be released, diffuse across the synapse, and bind to receptors
  - **Synaptic delay** - time needed to do this (0.3–5.0 ms) is the rate-limiting step of neural transmission

Figure 11.3 Chemical synapse

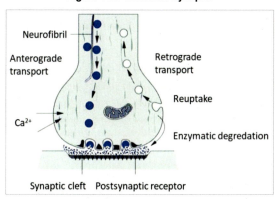

Postsynaptic Potentials
- **EPSP** - **e**xcitatory **p**ostsynaptic **p**otentials
- **IPSP** - **i**nhibitory **p**ostsynaptic **p**otentials
- **Excitatory Synapses and EPSPs**
  - Neurotransmitter binds to and opens chemically gated channels that allow simultaneous flow of Na^+ and K^+ in opposite directions
  - Na^+ influx is greater that K^+ efflux, causing a net **depolarization**
- **Inhibitory Synapses and IPSPs**
  - Neurotransmitter binds to and opens channels for K^+ or Cl^-
  - Causes a **hyperpolarization** (the inner surface of membrane becomes more negative)
  - Reduces the postsynaptic neuron's ability to produce an action potential
- **Summation** - A single EPSP cannot induce an action potential!

- EPSPs can summate to reach threshold; IPSPs can also summate with EPSPs, canceling each other out
  - **Temporal summation**: One or more presynaptic neurons transmit impulses in rapid-fire order
  - **Spatial summation**: Postsynaptic neuron is stimulated by a large number of terminals at the same time
- **Synaptic Potentiation**
  - Repeated use increases the efficiency of neurotransmission
  - Ca^{2+} concentration increases in presynaptic terminal and postsynaptic neuron
  - Brief high-frequency stimulation partially depolarizes the postsynaptic neuron
  - Chemically gated channels (**NMDA receptors**) allow Ca^{2+} entry
  - Ca^{2+} activates kinase enzymes that promote more effective responses to subsequent stimuli

Neurotransmitters
- **Chemical Classification**
  - **Acetylcholine** (Ach): Released at neuromuscular junctions and some ANS neurons; synthesized by choline acetyltransferase; degraded by **acetylcholinesterase** (AChE)
  - **Biogenic amines** include:
    - **Catecholamines**: Dopamine, norepinephrine (NE), and epinephrine
    - **Indolamines**: Serotonin and histamine
  - **Amino acids** include: GABA - Gamma (γ)-aminobutyric acid, glycine, aspartate, glutamate
  - **Peptides (neuropeptides)** include:
    - **Substance P**: Mediator of pain signals
    - **Endorphins**: Act as natural opiates; reduce pain perception
    - **Gut-brain peptides**: Somatostatin and cholecystokinin
  - **Purines** such as ATP act in both the CNS and PNS; produce fast or slow responses; induce Ca^{2+} influx in astrocytes; provoke pain sensation
  - **Gases and lipids**
    - **Nitric oxide** (NO) is involved in learning and memory
    - **Carbon monoxide** (CO) is a regulator of cGMP in the brain
  - **Endocannabinoids** are involved in learning and memory
- **Functional Classification**
  - Neurotransmitter effects may be **excitatory** (depolarizing) **and/or inhibitory** (hyperpolarizing)
  - **Determined by the receptor type** of the postsynaptic neuron
    - **Acetylcholine**
      - Excitatory at neuromuscular junctions in skeletal muscle
      - Inhibitory in cardiac muscle

Neurotransmitter Actions
- **Direct action**: Neurotransmitter binds to channel-linked receptor and opens ion channels; promotes rapid responses; e.g., ACh and amino acids
- **Indirect action**: Neurotransmitter binds to a G protein-linked receptor and acts through an intracellular second messenger; promotes long-lasting effects; e.g., biogenic amines, neuropeptides, and dissolved gases

A&P Essentials 4th ed.

Chapter 12 Central Nervous System

Central Nervous System (CNS) - brain and spinal cord

- **Adult brain regions**: Cerebral hemispheres, diencephalon, brain stem (midbrain, pons, and medulla); cerebellum
- **Ventricles of the Brain**
  - **Two** C-shaped **lateral ventricles** in the cerebral hemispheres
  - **Third ventricle** in the diencephalon
  - **Fourth ventricle** in the hindbrain, dorsal to the pons
  - Connected to one another and to the central canal of the spinal cord
  - Lined by **ependymal cells**
  - Contain **cerebrospinal fluid**
- **Spinal cord**
  - **Central cavity** surrounded by a **gray matter** core
  - External **white matter** composed of myelinated fiber tracts
- **Brain**
  - Similar pattern with additional areas of **gray matter**
  - **Nuclei** in cerebellum and cerebrum
  - **Cortex** of cerebellum and cerebrum

Figure 12.1 Regions of the brain

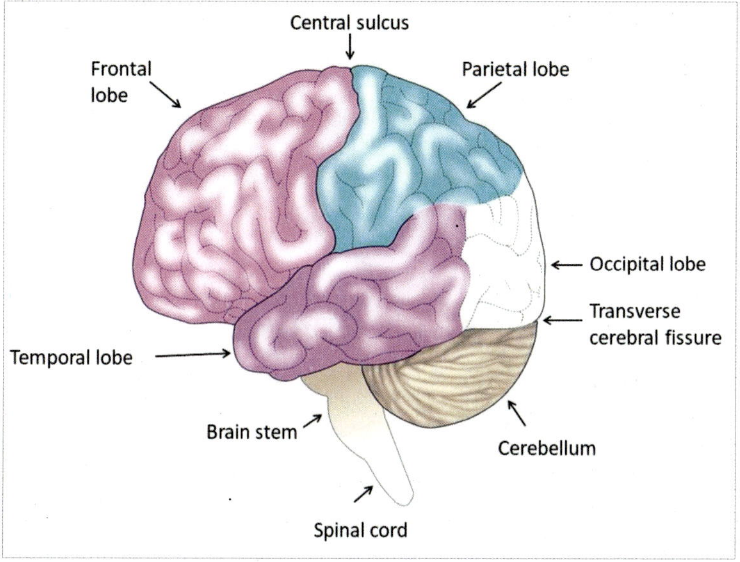

Labels: Central sulcus, Frontal lobe, Parietal lobe, Occipital lobe, Transverse cerebral fissure, Temporal lobe, Brain stem, Cerebellum, Spinal cord

Cerebral Hemispheres

- **Five lobes**: frontal, parietal, temporal, occipital, insula
- **Central sulcus**: Separates the precentral gyrus of the frontal lobe and the postcentral gyrus of the parietal lobe
- **Longitudinal fissure**: Separates the two hemispheres
- **Transverse cerebral fissure**: Separates the cerebrum and the cerebellum

Cerebral Cortex

- Thin (2–4 mm) superficial layer of **gray matter**; 40% of the mass of the brain
- **Site of conscious mind**: awareness, sensory perception, voluntary motor initiation, communication, memory storage, understanding
- Each hemisphere connects to contralateral side of the body
- **Three functional areas (SAM)**
  - **Sensory areas** - conscious awareness of sensation
  - **Association areas** - integrate diverse information
  - **Motor areas** - control voluntary movement
- Conscious behavior involves the entire cortex

Sensory Areas

- **Primary Somatosensory Cortex**: In the postcentral gyri; receives sensory information from the skin, skeletal muscles, and joints; capable of spatial discrimination: identification of body region being stimulated
- **Somatosensory Association Cortex**: Integrates sensory input from primary somatosensory cortex; determines size, texture, and relationship of parts of objects being felt
- **Visual Areas**
  - **Primary visual (striate) cortex**: Extreme posterior tip of the occipital lobe; receives visual information from the retinas
  - **Visual association area**: Surrounds the primary visual cortex; uses past visual experiences to interpret visual stimuli; complex processing involves entire posterior half of the hemispheres
- **Auditory Areas**
  - **Primary auditory cortex**: Interprets information from inner ear as pitch, loudness, and location
  - **Auditory association area**: Stores memories of sounds and permits perception of sounds
- **Olfactory Cortex**: Region of conscious awareness of odors
- **Gustatory Cortex**: Involved in the perception of taste
- **Visceral Sensory Area**: Conscious perception of visceral sensations
- **Vestibular Cortex**: Responsible for conscious awareness of balance (position of the head in space)

- **Multimodal Association Areas** - Receive inputs from multiple sensory areas
  - Send outputs to multiple areas, including the premotor cortex
  - Allow us to give meaning to information received, store it as memory, compare it to previous experience, and decide on action to take
  - **Anterior Association Area (Prefrontal Cortex)**: Most complicated cortical region
    - Involved with intellect, cognition, recall, and personality
    - Contains working memory for judgment, reasoning, persistence, and conscience
    - Development depends on feedback from social environment
  - **Posterior Association Area**: Large region in temporal, parietal, and occipital lobes
    - Plays a role in recognizing patterns and faces and localizing us in space
    - Involved in understanding written and spoken language (**Wernicke's area**)
  - **Limbic Association Area**: Provides emotional impact that helps establish memories

Motor Areas
- **Primary (somatic) motor cortex**: Large pyramidal cells of the precentral gyri; long axons → pyramidal (corticospinal) tracts
- Allows conscious control of precise, skilled, voluntary movements
- **Motor homunculus**: upside-down caricature representing the motor innervation of body regions
- **Premotor cortex**: Anterior to the precentral gyrus; controls learned, repetitious, or patterned motor skills
- Coordinates simultaneous or sequential actions
- Involved in the planning of movements that depend on sensory feedback
- **Broca's area**: Motor speech area that directs muscles of the tongue; present in one hemisphere (usually the left)
- **Frontal eye field**: Controls voluntary eye movements

Lateralization of Cortical Function: Division of labor between hemispheres
- **Cerebral dominance**: Designates the hemisphere dominant for language (left hemisphere in 90% of people)
  - **Left hemisphere**: Controls language, math, and logic
  - **Right hemisphere**: Insight, visual-spatial skills, intuition, and artistic skills
- Left and right hemispheres communicate via fiber tracts in the cerebral white matter

Cerebral White Matter
- Myelinated fibers and their tracts responsible for communication
- **Commissures** (in corpus callosum) - connect gray matter of the two hemispheres
- **Association fibers** - connect different parts of the same hemisphere
- **Projection fibers** - (corona radiata) connect the hemispheres with lower brain or spinal cord

Basal Nuclei
- Subcortical nuclei; consists of the **corpus striatum** (caudate nucleus; lentiform nucleus)
- Influence muscular control
- Help regulate attention and cognition
- Regulate intensity of slow or stereotyped movements
- Inhibit antagonistic and unnecessary movements

Diencephalon

Thalamus: 80% of diencephalon
- Connected by the **interthalamic adhesion** (intermediate mass)
- Nuclei project and receive fibers from the cerebral cortex
- **Function** - Gateway to the cerebral cortex; sorts, edits, and relays information
- Mediates sensation, motor activities, cortical arousal, learning, and memory

Hypothalamus: Forms the inferolateral walls of the third ventricle
- **Infundibulum** - stalk that connects to the pituitary gland
- Autonomic control center for many visceral functions
- **Center for emotional response**: Involved in perception of pleasure, fear, and rage

and in biological rhythms and drives
- Regulates body temperature, food intake, water balance, and thirst
- Regulates sleep and the sleep cycle
- Controls release of hormones by the anterior pituitary
- Produces posterior pituitary hormones
- **Epithalamus**: Most dorsal portion of the diencephalon; forms roof of the third ventricle
  - **Pineal gland** - extends from the posterior border and secretes **melatonin** (helps regulate sleep-wake cycles)

Brain Stem

- Similar structure to spinal cord; contains embedded nuclei
- Controls automatic behaviors necessary for survival
- Contains fiber tracts connecting higher and lower neural centers

Midbrain - Located between the diencephalon and the pons
- **Cerebral peduncles**: Contain pyramidal motor tracts
- **Cerebral aqueduct**: Channel between third and fourth ventricles
- **Nuclei** that control cranial nerves III (oculomotor) and IV (trochlear)

Pons - Forms part of the anterior wall of the fourth ventricle
- Fibers of the pons connect higher brain centers and the spinal cord; relay impulses between the motor cortex and the cerebellum
- Origin of cranial nerves V (trigeminal), VI (abducens), and VII (facial)
- Some nuclei of the reticular formation
- Nuclei that help maintain normal rhythm of breathing

Medulla Oblongata - Joins spinal cord at foramen magnum
- **Pyramids** - two ventral longitudinal ridges formed by pyramidal tracts
  - **Decussation of the pyramids** - crossover of the corticospinal tracts
- Cranial nerves VIII, X, and XII are associated with the medulla
- Vestibular nuclear complex - mediates responses that maintain equilibrium
- **Cardiovascular center** adjusts force and rate of heart contraction and blood vessel diameter for blood pressure regulation
- **Respiratory centers** generate respiratory rhythm and control rate and depth of breathing
- **Additional centers** regulate vomiting, hiccupping, swallowing, coughing, sneezing

Cerebellum

- Dorsal to pons and medulla; 11% of brain mass
- Subconsciously provides precise timing and appropriate patterns of skeletal muscle contraction
- **Two hemispheres** connected by **vermis**; each hemisphere has three **lobes** (anterior, posterior, and flocculonodular)
  - **Folia** - Transversely oriented gyri
  - **Arbor vitae** - Distinctive treelike pattern of the cerebellar white matter
  - **Cerebellar Peduncles** - Three paired fiber tracts connect cerebellum to brain stem
- **Cerebellar Processing for Motor Activity**
  - Cerebellum receives impulses from the cerebral cortex of the intent to initiate volun-

- tary muscle contraction
  - Signals from proprioceptors and visual and equilibrium pathways continuously "inform" the cerebellum of the body's position and momentum
  - **Cerebellar cortex** calculates the best way to smoothly coordinate a muscle contraction; a "blueprint" of coordinated movement is sent to the cerebral motor cortex and to brain stem nuclei
- **Cognitive Function of the Cerebellum**
  - Recognizes and predicts sequences of events during complex movements
  - Plays a role in nonmotor functions such as word association and puzzle solving

Functional Brain Systems

- Networks of neurons that work together and span wide areas of the brain
- **Limbic System** - Emotional or affective brain
  - Includes parts of the diencephalon and some cerebral structures that encircle the brain stem
  - **Amygdala** - recognizes angry or fearful facial expressions, assesses danger, and elicits the fear response
  - **Cingulate gyrus** - plays a role in expressing emotions via gestures, and resolves mental conflict
  - Puts emotional responses to odors
  - **Hippocampus** and **amygdala** - play a role in memory
- **Reticular Formation**
  - Three broad columns along the length of the brain stem
  - Has far-flung axonal connections with hypothalamus, thalamus, cerebral cortex, cerebellum, and spinal cord
- **RAS (reticular activating system)**
  - Sends impulses to the cerebral cortex to keep it conscious and alert
  - Filters out repetitive and weak stimuli (~99% of all stimuli!)
  - Severe injury results in permanent unconsciousness (coma)
- **Motor function**
  - Helps control coarse limb movements
  - Reticular autonomic centers regulate visceral motor functions
    - Vasomotor
    - Cardiac
    - Respiratory centers

Memory

- Storage and retrieval of information
- **Short-term memory** (STM, or working memory) - temporary holding of information; limited to seven or eight pieces of information
- **Long-term memory** (LTM) has limitless capacity
  - **Transfer from STM to LTM**
    - Factors that affect transfer from STM to LTM
      - **Emotional state** - best if alert, motivated, surprised, and aroused
      - **Rehearsal** - repetition and practice
      - **Association** - tying new information with old memories

- **Automatic memory** - subconscious information stored in LTM
- **Declarative memory** (**factual knowledge**) - Explicit information
  - Related to our conscious thoughts and our language ability
  - Stored in LTM with context in which it was learned
- **Nondeclarative memory** - Best remembered by doing; hard to unlearn
  - Less conscious or unconscious
  - Acquired through experience and repetition
  - Includes procedural (skills) memory, motor memory, and emotional memory

Sleep

- State of partial unconsciousness from which a person can be aroused by stimulation
- Two major types of sleep (defined by EEG patterns)
  - **Nonrapid eye movement** (NREM)
  - **Rapid eye movement** (REM)
- Alternating cycles of sleep and wakefulness reflect a natural **circadian** (24-hour) **rhythm**
- RAS activity is inhibited during, but RAS also mediates, dreaming sleep
- A typical sleep pattern alternates between REM and NREM sleep
- **Importance of Sleep**
  - Slow-wave sleep (NREM stages 3 and 4) is presumed to be the restorative stage
  - People deprived of REM sleep become moody and depressed
  - REM sleep may be a reverse learning process where superfluous information is purged from the brain
  - Daily sleep requirements decline with age; stage 4 sleep declines steadily and may disappear after age 60

Spinal Cord

- Begins at the foramen magnum - Ends as **conus medullaris** at L_1 vertebra
- Provides two-way communication to and from the brain
- Contains spinal reflex centers
- **Spinal nerves** - 31 pairs
- **Cervical and lumbar enlargements**: The nerves serving the upper and lower limbs emerge here
- **Cauda equina**: The collection of nerve roots at the inferior end of the vertebral canal
- **Cross-Sectional Anatomy**
  - Two lengthwise **grooves** divide cord into right and left halves
    - **Ventral** (anterior) **median fissure**
    - **Dorsal** (posterior) **median sulcus**
  - **Gray commissure** - connects masses of gray matter; encloses central canal

Gray Matter
- **Dorsal horns** - interneurons that receive somatic and visceral sensory input
- **Ventral horns** - somatic motor neurons whose axons exit the cord via ventral roots
- **Lateral horns** (only in thoracic and lumbar regions) –sympathetic neurons
- **Dorsal root (spinal) ganglia** - contain cell bodies of sensory neurons

White Matter - Consists mostly of ascending (sensory) and descending (motor) tracts

A&P Essentials 4th ed.

- Transverse tracts (commissural fibers) cross from one side to the other
- **Pathway Generalizations**
  - Pathways decussate (cross over)
  - Pathways are paired symmetrically (one on each side of the spinal cord or brain)
- **Ascending Pathways**
  - Two pathways transmit somatosensory information to the sensory cortex via the thalamus
    - **Dorsal column-medial lemniscal pathways**: Transmit input to the somatosensory cortex for discriminative touch and vibrations
    - **Spinothalamic pathways**: Transmit pain, temperature, and coarse touch impulses within the lateral spinothalamic tract
  - **Spinocerebellar tracts** terminate in the cerebellum; Convey information about muscle or tendon stretch to the cerebellum
- **Descending Pathways and Tracts** - Deliver efferent impulses from the brain to the spinal cord
  - Innervate skeletal muscles
- **Direct pathways** - Direct (Pyramidal) System
  - Regulates fast and fine (skilled) movements
- **Indirect pathways** - Indirect (Extrapyramidal) System
  - Includes the brain stem motor nuclei, and all motor pathways except pyramidal pathways
  - These pathways are complex and multisynaptic, and **regulate**:
    - Axial muscles that maintain balance and posture
    - Muscles controlling coarse movements
    - Head, neck, and eye movements that follow objects

Figure 12.2 Spinal cord, cross section

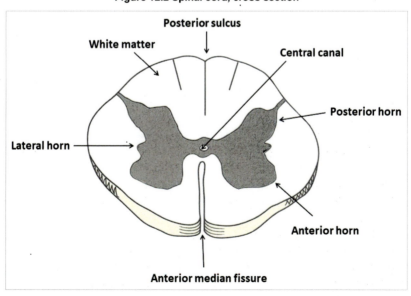

Protection of the Brain and Spinal Chord

Bone (skull) – see **Chapter 7 Skeleton**

Meninges - Cover and protect the CNS
- Protect blood vessels and enclose venous sinuses
- Contain cerebrospinal fluid (CSF)
- **Dura Mater** - Strongest meninx
  - Two layers of fibrous connective tissue (around the brain) separate to form dural sinuses
  - Dural septa limit excessive movement of the brain
    - **Falx cerebri** - in the longitudinal fissure; attached to **crista galli**
    - **Falx cerebelli** - along the vermis of the cerebellum
    - **Tentorium cerebelli** - horizontal dural fold over cerebellum and in the transverse fissure
- **Arachnoid Mater** - Middle layer with weblike extensions
  - Separated from the dura mater by the **subdural space**
  - **Subarachnoid space** contains CSF and blood vessels
  - **Arachnoid villi** protrude into the superior sagittal sinus and permit CSF reabsorption
- **Pia Mater** - Layer of delicate vascularized connective tissue that clings tightly to the brain

Cerebrospinal Fluid (CSF)
- **Composition**: Watery solution; less protein and different ion concentrations than plasma; constant volume
- **Functions**: Gives buoyancy to the CNS organs; protects the CNS from blows and other trauma; nourishes the brain and carries chemical signals
- **Choroid Plexuses** - Produce CSF at a constant rate
  - Hang from the roof of each ventricle
  - Clusters of capillaries enclosed by pia mater and a layer of **ependymal cells**

Blood-Brain Barrier
- Feet of astrocytes provide signal to endothelium for the formation of tight junctions
- Helps maintain a stable environment for the brain
- Allows nutrients to move by facilitated diffusion
- Allows any fat-soluble substances to pass, including alcohol, nicotine, and anesthetics
- Absent in some areas, e.g., vomiting center and the hypothalamus, where it is necessary to monitor the chemical composition of the blood

Protection of the Spinal Cord
- Bone, meninges, and CSF
- Cushion of fat and a network of veins in the epidural space between the vertebrae and spinal dura mater
- CSF in subarachnoid space
- **Denticulate ligaments**: extensions of pia mater that secure cord to dura mater
- **Filum terminale**: fibrous extension from conus medullaris; anchors the spinal cord to the coccyx

Chapter 13 Peripheral Nervous System & Reflexes

Peripheral Nervous System (PNS)

- **All neural structures outside the brain**
  - Sensory receptors
  - Peripheral nerves and associated ganglia
  - Motor endings

Nerves - Bundle of myelinated and unmyelinated peripheral axons enclosed by connective tissue
- **Endoneurium** - loose connective tissue that encloses axons and their myelin sheaths
- **Perineurium** - coarse connective tissue that bundles fibers into fascicles
- **Epineurium** - tough fibrous sheath around a nerve

Classification of Nerves
- Most nerves are mixtures of afferent and efferent fibers and somatic and autonomic (visceral) fibers
- Pure **sensory** (afferent) or **motor** (efferent) **nerves** are rare
- Types of fibers in **mixed nerves**:
  - Somatic afferent and somatic efferent
  - Visceral afferent and visceral efferent
- Peripheral nerves classified as **cranial** or **spinal nerves**

Ganglia - Contain neuron cell bodies associated with nerves
- **Dorsal root ganglia** (sensory, somatic)
- **Autonomic ganglia** (motor, visceral)

Regeneration of nerve fibers
- If the soma of a damaged nerve is intact, axon will regenerate
- Involves coordinated activity among:
  - **Macrophages** - remove debris
  - **Schwann cells** - form regeneration tube and secrete growth factors
  - **Axons** - regenerate damaged part
- CNS **oligodendrocytes** bear growth-inhibiting proteins that **prevent CNS fiber regeneration**

Cranial Nerves
- Twelve pairs of nerves associated with the brain
- Most are mixed in function; two pairs (CN I & II) are purely sensory

Nerve	Components	Main action
Olfactory nerve (I)	Special sensory	Smell sensation
Optic nerve (II)	Special sensory	Visual signals from retina
Oculomotor nerve (III)	Somatic motor	Superior, inferior and medial rectus, inferior oblique and levator palpebrae inferioris muscle
	Visceral motor (Parasympathetic)	Sphincter pupillae and ciliary muscles
Trochlear nerve (IV)	Somatic motor	Superior oblique muscle

Trigeminal nerve (V)		
Ophthalmic nerve	General sensory	Cornea, skin of forehead, scalp, eyelids and nose, and mucosa of nasal cavity and paranasal sinuses
Maxillary nerve	General sensory	Skin of face over maxilla, upper lip, maxillary teeth, mucosa of nose, maxillary sinus and palate
Mandibular nerve	General sensory	Skin over mandible, lower lip, mandibular teeth, temporomandibular joint, mucosa of mouth and anterior 2/3 of tongue
	Somatic motor	Muscles of mastication, mylohyoid, anterior belly of digastric, tensor veli palatini and tensor tympani muscle
Abducent nerve (VI)	Somatic motor	Lateral rectus muscle
Facial nerve (VII)	Somatic motor	Muscles of facial expression and scalp, stapedius, stylohyoid and posterior belly of digastric muscle
	Special sensory	Taste from anterior 2/3 of tongue, floor of mouth and palate
	General sensory	Skin of external acoustic meatus
	Visceral motor (Parasympathetic)	Submandibular and sublingual glands, lacrimal gland, glands of nose and palate
Vestibulocochlear nerve (VIII)		
Vestibular nerve	Special sensory	Vestibular signals from semicircular ducts, utricle and saccule
Cochlear nerve	Special sensory	Auditory signals from Corti organ in cochlea
Glossopharyngeal nerve (IX)	Somatic motor	Stylopharyngeus muscle
	Visceral motor (Parasympathetic)	Parotid gland
	Visceral sensory	Parotid gland, carotid body and sinus, pharynx and middle ear
	Special sensory	Taste from posterior 1/3 of tongue
	General sensory	Skin of external ear
Vagus nerve (X)	Somatic motor	Constrictor muscles of pharynx, intrinsic muscles of larynx, muscles of palate, striated muscles upper 2/3 of esophagus
	Visceral motor (Parasympathetic)	Trachea, bronchi and digestive tract; sinoatrial and atrioventricular node of heart
	Special sensory	Taste from epiglottis and palate

	Visceral sensory	Base of tongue, pharynx, larynx, trachea, bronchi, heart, esophagus, stomach and intestines
	General sensory	Skin of auricle, external acoustic meatus and dura mater of posterior cranial fossa
Accessory nerve (XI)	Somatic motor	Sternocleidomastoid and trapezius muscle
Hypoglossal nerve (XII)	Somatic motor	Muscles of tongue (except palatoglossus)

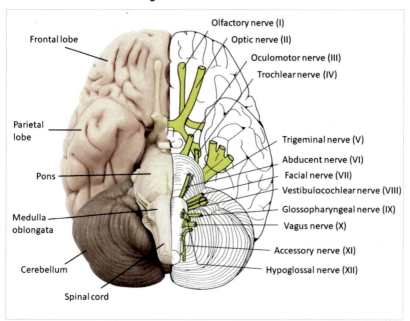

Figure 13.1 Cranial nerves

Spinal Nerves

31 pairs of mixed nerves named according to their point of issue from the spinal cord
- 8 cervical (C_1–C_8)
- 12 thoracic (T_1–T_{12})
- 5 Lumbar (L_1–L_5)
- 5 Sacral (S_1–S_5)
- 1 Coccygeal (C_0)

Roots - Each spinal nerve connects to the spinal cord via two roots
- **Ventral roots**: Motor (efferent) fibers from ventral horn motor neurons to skeletal muscles
- **Dorsal roots**: Sensory (afferent) fibers from sensory neurons in the dorsal root ganglia; conduct impulses from peripheral receptors
- **Dorsal and ventral roots unite to form spinal nerves**, which then emerge from the

vertebral column via the intervertebral foramina

Rami - Each spinal nerve branches into mixed rami
- **Dorsal ramus**
- Larger **ventral ramus**
- **Meningeal branch**
- **Rami communicantes** (autonomic pathways) join to the ventral rami in the thoracic region
  - All **ventral rami except T_2–T_{12} form** interlacing nerve networks called **plexuses** (cervical, brachial, lumbar, and sacral)
  - The **back** is innervated by **dorsal rami** via several branches
  - **Ventral rami of T_2–T_{12}** as **intercostal nerves** supply muscles of the ribs, anterolateral thorax, and abdominal wall

- **Innervation of Skin**
  - **Dermatome**: the area of skin innervated by the cutaneous branches of a single spinal nerve; all spinal nerves except C_1 participate in dermatomes
    - Most dermatomes overlap, so destruction of a single spinal nerve will not cause complete numbness
- **Innervation of Joints**
  - **Hilton's law**: Any nerve serving a muscle that produces movement at a joint also innervates the joint and the skin over the joint

Spinal plexuses and major nerves

Cervical plexus [C_1-C_4] - Innervates skin and muscles of neck, ear, back of head, and shoulders

Phrenic nerve	Diaphragm

Brachial plexus [C_5-T_1; (C_4) –(T_2)] - Gives rise to nerves that innervate the upper limb

Musculocutaneous nerve	Flexor muscles of arm (biceps brachii, brachialis, coracobrachialis)
	Skin of lateral forearm
Median nerve	Flexors of anterior forearm (flexor carpi radialis, flexor digitorum superficialis, flexor pollicis longus, palmaris longus lateral part of flexor digitorum profundus, pronator teres and quadratus); intrinsic muscles of lateral palm and digital branches to fingers
	Skin of lateral 2/3 of hand, palm side and dorsum of fingers 2-3
Ulnar nerve	Flexor muscles in anterior forearm (flexor carpi ulnaris, medial part of flexor digitorum profundus); most intrinsic hand muscles
	Skin of anterior and posterior medial third of hand
Radial nerve	Posterior muscles of arm and forearm (brachioradialis, triceps brachii, anconeus, supinator, all extensor muscles and abductor pollicis longus)
	Skin of posterolateral surface of entire upper limb except dorsum of fingers 2-3

Axillary nerve	Deltoid and teres minor Skin of shoulder region over deltoid
Lumbar plexus [L₁ –L₄] - Innervates thigh, abdominal wall, and psoas muscle	
Femoral nerve	Anterior muscles of thigh (quadriceps, Sartorius), pectineus and iliacus Skin of anterior and medial thigh, medial leg and foot, hip and knee join
Obturator nerve	Adductor magnus, longus and brevis, gracilis and obturator externus Skin of medial thigh, hip and knee joint
Sacral plexus [L₄ –S₄] - Innervates buttock, lower limb, pelvic structures, and perineum	
Sciatic nerve	
Tibial nerve	Hamstrings, adductor magnus (posterior part), triceps surae, tibialis posterior, popliteus, flexor digitorum longus, flexor halluces longus and intrinsic foot muscle Skin of posterior surface of leg and sole of foot
Common fibular nerve	Short head of biceps femoris, fibularis longus, brevis and tertius, tibialis anterior, extensor digitorum longus and extensor hallucis longus Skin of anterior and lateral surface of leg and top of foot

Autonomic Nervous System

- Consists of motor neurons that:
  - Innervate smooth and cardiac muscle and glands
  - Make adjustments to ensure optimal support for body activities
  - Operate via subconscious control

Divisions of the ANS

Parasympathetic Division
- Promotes maintenance activities and conserves body energy
- **Rest-and-relaxation division**
  - Blood pressure, heart rate, and respiratory rates are low
  - Gastrointestinal tract activity is high
  - Pupils are constricted and lenses are accommodated for close vision
- Because its preganglionic neurons are located in the brain and the sacral spinal cord it is sometimes called the **craniosacral division**.
- **Cranial nerve X** (aka **vagus nerve**) carries 90% of all parasympathetic fibers to organs in the abdominal cavity.
- At rest the body is under a parasympathetic tone. The parasympathetic system normally dominates the heart and smooth muscle of digestive and urinary tract organs.
  - Slows the heart
  - Dictates normal activity levels of the digestive and urinary tracts
  - The sympathetic division can override these effects during times of stress

Sympathetic (Thoracolumbar) Division
- Promotes adjustments during exercise, or when threatened

- **Fight-or-flight system**
  - Blood flow is shunted to skeletal muscles and heart
  - Bronchioles dilate
  - Liver releases glucose
- **Preganglionic neurons** are in spinal cord segments $T_1 - L_2$
- Sympathetic neurons produce the lateral horns of the spinal cord
- Preganglionic fibers pass through the white rami communicantes and enter **sympathetic trunk** (paravertebral) **ganglia**
- There are 23 paravertebral ganglia in the sympathetic trunk (chain)
  - Upon entering a sympathetic trunk ganglion a preganglionic fiber may:
  - Synapse with a ganglionic neuron within the same ganglion
  - Ascend or descend the sympathetic trunk to synapse in another trunk ganglion
  - Pass through the trunk ganglion and emerge without synapsing
- **Unique Roles of the Sympathetic Division**
  - The adrenal medulla, sweat glands, arrector pili muscles, kidneys, and most blood vessels receive only sympathetic fibers

Dual innervation - Almost all visceral organs are served by both divisions, but they cause opposite effects
- **Cooperative Effects - Best seen in control of the external genitalia**
  - **Parasympathetic fibers** cause vasodilation; are responsible for erection of the penis or clitoris
  - **Sympathetic fibers** cause ejaculation of semen in males and reflex contraction of a female's vagina

Table 13.1 Effects of sympathetic and parasympathetic stimulation on various organ systems

Organ (system)	Sympathetic stimulation	Parasympathetic stimulation
Cardiovascular system		
Heart muscle	Increased heart rate Increased contractility	Decreased heart rate Decreased contractility (esp. atria)
Lungs		
Bronchi	Dilation	Constriction
Skin		
Blood vessels	Constriction	None
Arrector pili muscles	Contraction	None
Digestive system		
Salivary glands, exocrine pancreas and gastric glands	Vasoconstriction and slight secretion	Copious secretion
Liver	Release of glucose	Slight glycogen synthesis
Gallbladder and bile ducts	Relaxation	Contraction
Small and large intestine	Decreased peristalsis;	Increased peristalsis; re-

	increased sphincter tone	laxed sphincter tone
Urinary & reproductive system		
Kidneys	Decreased urine production	None
Penis	Ejaculation	Erection
Eyes		
Pupil	Dilation	Constriction
Ciliary muscle	Slight relaxation (far vision)	Constriction (near vision)
Endocrine system/metabolism		
Basal metabolism	Increased up to 100%	None
Adrenal medulla	Increased secretion	None
Fat tissue	Increased breakdown of fat	None
Mental activity	Increased	None

Pathways of the ANS

Efferent Pathway is a two-neuron chain
- **Preganglionic neuron** (in CNS) has a thin, lightly myelinated preganglionic axon
- **Ganglionic neuron** in autonomic ganglion has an unmyelinated **postganglionic axon** that extends to the effector organ

Neurotransmitter Effects
- **Preganglionic fibers** release **ACh**
- **Postganglionic fibers** release **norepinephrine** or **Ach**
- Effect is either stimulatory or inhibitory, depending on type of receptors

Neurotransmitters and Receptors

- **Cholinergic fibers** release the neurotransmitter **ACh**
  - All ANS preganglionic axons
  - All parasympathetic postganglionic axons
- **Adrenergic fibers** release the neurotransmitter **NE**
  - Most sympathetic postganglionic axons; **exceptions**: sympathetic postganglionic fibers secrete ACh at sweat glands and some blood vessels in skeletal muscles
- **Cholinergic Receptors bind ACh**
  - **Nicotinic Receptors**
    - Motor end plates of skeletal muscle cells
    - All ganglionic neurons (sympathetic and parasympathetic)
    - Hormone-producing cells of the adrenal medulla
    - Effect of ACh at **nicotinic receptors** is **always stimulatory**
  - **Muscarinic Receptors**
    - All effector cells stimulated by postganglionic cholinergic fibers
    - The **effect** of ACh at muscarinic receptors can be **either inhibitory or excitatory** depending on the receptor type of the target organ
- **Adrenergic Receptors bind NE**
  - **Alpha** (α) (subtypes α_1, α_2)

- **Beta** (β) (subtypes β₁, β₂, β₃)
- Effects of NE depend on which subclass of receptor predominates on the target organ
- **Parasympathetic division**: short-lived, highly localized control over effectors
- **Sympathetic division**: long-lasting, bodywide effects
- Long lasting because NE is inactivated more slowly than ACh
- **NE and epinephrine are released into the blood and remain there until destroyed by the liver**

Control of ANS Function

- **Hypothalamus** - main integrative center of ANS activity
- **Subconscious cerebral** input via limbic lobe connections influences hypothalamic function
- Other controls come from the cerebral cortex, the reticular formation, and the spinal cord
- **Hypothalamic Control** - Direct or indirect (through the reticular system)
  - Heart activity and blood pressure
  - Body temperature, water balance, and endocrine activity
  - Emotional stages (rage, pleasure) and biological drives (hunger, thirst, sex)
  - Reactions to fear and the "fight-or-flight" system

Reflexes

- **Inborn (intrinsic) reflex**: a rapid, involuntary, predictable motor response to a stimulus
- **Learned (acquired) reflexes** result from practice or repetition, e.g., driving skills
- Components of a **reflex arc** (neural path)
  - **Receptor** - site of stimulus action
  - **Sensory neuron** - transmits afferent impulses to the CNS
  - **Integration center** - either monosynaptic or polysynaptic region within the CNS
  - **Motor neuron** - conducts efferent impulses from the integration center to an effector organ
  - Effector - **muscle fiber or gland cell that responds to the efferent impulses by contracting or secreting**

Spinal (somatic) Reflexes

- Integration center is in the spinal cord
- Effectors are skeletal muscle
- Testing of somatic reflexes is important clinically to assess the condition of the nervous system

Stretch and Golgi Tendon Reflexes

- For skeletal muscle activity to be smoothly coordinated, proprioceptor input is necessary
  - **Muscle spindles** inform the nervous system of the length of the muscle
  - **Golgi tendon organs** inform the brain as to the amount of tension in the muscle and tendons
- **Stretch Reflexes** - Maintain muscle tone in large postural muscles

- **Cause muscle contraction in response to increased muscle length** (stretch)
- Stretch activates the muscle spindle
- Sensory neurons synapse directly with motor neurons in the spinal cord
- Motor neurons cause the stretched muscle to contract
- All stretch reflexes are **monosynaptic** and **ipsilateral**
- **Reciprocal inhibition** also occurs; e.g., in the patellar reflex, the stretched muscle (quadriceps) contracts and the antagonists (hamstrings) relax
- **Golgi Tendon Reflexes** - Help to prevent damage due to excessive stretch
- Polysynaptic reflexes
- Important for smooth onset and termination of muscle contraction
- Produce **muscle relaxation (lengthening) in response to tension**
- Contraction or passive stretch activates Golgi tendon organs → afferent impulses are transmitted to spinal cord → contracting muscle relaxes and the antagonist contracts (**reciprocal activation**)
- Information transmitted simultaneously to the cerebellum is used to adjust muscle tension

Flexor and Crossed-Extensor Reflexes
- **Flexor (withdrawal) reflex** - Causes automatic withdrawal of the threatened body part
  - Initiated by a painful stimulus
  - **Ipsilateral** and **polysynaptic**
- **Crossed extensor reflex** - Occurs with flexor reflexes in weight-bearing limbs to maintain balance
  - Consists of an ipsilateral flexor reflex and a contralateral extensor reflex
  - The stimulated side is withdrawn (flexed)
  - The contralateral side is extended

Superficial Reflexes - Elicited by gentle cutaneous stimulation
- Depend on upper motor pathways and cord-level reflex arcs
- **Plantar** reflex
  - **Stimulus**: stroking lateral aspect of the sole of the foot
  - **Response**: downward flexion of the toes
  - Tests for function of corticospinal tracts

- **Babinski sign**
  - **Stimulus**: as above
  - **Response**: dorsiflexion of hallux and fanning of toes
  - Present in infants due to incomplete myelination
  - In adults, indicates corticospinal or motor cortex damage

- **Abdominal reflexes**
  - Cause contraction of abdominal muscles and movement of the umbilicus in response to stroking of the skin
  - Vary in intensity from one person to another
  - Absent when corticospinal tract lesions are present

Visceral Reflexes
- Have the same components as somatic reflexes
- Visceral pain afferents travel along the same pathways as somatic pain fibers, contributing to the phenomenon of referred pain

- Visceral pain afferents travel along the same pathway as somatic pain fibers
- Pain stimuli arising in the viscera are perceived as somatic in origin

A&P Essentials 4th ed.

Chapter 14 General & Special Senses

From Sensation to Perception

- **Sensation**: the awareness of changes in the internal and external environment
- **Perception**: the conscious interpretation of stimuli

Sensory Integration
- Input from exteroceptors, proprioceptors, and interoceptors is relayed toward the head, but is processed along the way
- Processing at the Receptor Level
  - Receptors have **specificity** for stimulus energy
  - Stimulus must be applied in a **receptive field**
  - Stimulus energy is converted into a graded potential called a **receptor potential**
  - Adaptation is a change in sensitivity in the presence of a constant stimulus
    - **Phasic (fast-adapting) receptors** signal the beginning or end of a stimulus; e.g., receptors for pressure, touch, and smell
    - **Tonic receptors** adapt slowly or not at all; e.g., nociceptors
- Processing at the Circuit Level
- Pathways of three neurons conduct sensory impulses upward to the appropriate brain regions
  - **First-order neurons**: Receptor → CNS
  - **Second-order neurons**: Transmit impulses to the thalamus or cerebellum
  - **Third-order neurons**: Thalamus → somatosensory cortex (perceptual level)
- Processing at the Perceptual Level
  - Identification of the sensation depends on the specific location of the target neurons in the sensory cortex
    - **Perceptual detection** - ability to detect a stimulus
    - **Magnitude estimation** - intensity is coded in the frequency of impulses
    - **Spatial discrimination** - identifying the site or pattern of the stimulus

Main Aspects of Sensory Perception
- **Feature abstraction** - identification of more complex aspects and several stimulus properties
- **Quality discrimination** - the ability to identify submodalities of a sensation
- **Pattern recognition** - recognition of familiar or significant patterns in stimuli

Perception of Pain
- **Warns of actual or impending tissue damage**
- Stimuli include extreme pressure and temperature, histamine, K^+, ATP, acids, and bradykinin
- Impulses travel on fibers that release neurotransmitters glutamate and substance P
- Some pain impulses are blocked by inhibitory endogenous opioids

Sensory Receptors

- Specialized to respond to changes in their environment (stimuli)
- Activation results in graded potentials that trigger nerve impulses
- **Sensation** (awareness of stimulus) **and perception** (interpretation of the meaning of the stimulus) **occur in the brain**

Classification by Stimulus Type
- **Mechanoreceptors** - respond to touch, pressure, vibration, stretch, and itch
- **Thermoreceptors** - sensitive to changes in temperature
- **Photoreceptors** - respond to light energy (e.g., retina)
- **Chemoreceptors** - respond to chemicals (e.g., smell, changes in blood chemistry)
- **Nociceptors** - sensitive to pain-causing stimuli (e.g. extreme heat or cold)

Classification by Location
- **Exteroceptors** - Respond to stimuli arising outside the body; receptors in the skin for touch, pressure, pain, and temperature; most special sense organs
- **Interoceptors** (visceroceptors) - Respond to stimuli arising in internal organs and blood vessels; sensitive to chemical changes, tissue stretch, and temperature changes
- **Proprioceptors** - Respond to stretch in skeletal muscles, tendons, joints, ligaments, and connective tissue coverings of bones and muscles; inform the brain of the body's movements

Classification by Structural Complexity
- **Complex receptors (special sense organs)**: Vision, hearing, equilibrium, smell, and taste
- **Simple receptors for general senses**: Tactile sensations (touch, pressure, stretch, vibration), temperature, pain, and muscle sense
- **Unencapsulated Dendritic Endings**
  - **Thermoreceptors**
    - **Cold receptors** (50–104°F); in superficial dermis
    - **Heat receptors** (90–120°F); in deeper dermis
  - **Nociceptors** respond to pinching, chemicals from damaged tissue, temperatures outside the range of thermoreceptors, capsaicin
  - **Light touch receptors**
    - Tactile (Merkel) discs
    - Hair follicle receptors
- **Encapsulated Dendritic Endings** - All are mechanoreceptors
  - **Meissner's (tactile) corpuscles** - discriminative touch
  - **Pacinian (lamellated) corpuscles** - deep pressure and vibration
  - **Ruffini endings** - deep continuous pressure
  - **Muscle spindles** - muscle stretch
  - **Golgi tendon organs** - stretch in tendons
  - **Joint kinesthetic receptors** - stretch in joint capsules

Eye and Vision

- 70% of all sensory receptors are in the eye
- Nearly half of the cerebral cortex is involved in processing visual information!

Accessory Structures of the Eye - Protect the eye and aid eye function
- **Eyebrows** - Overlie the supraorbital margins; shade the eye; prevent perspiration from reaching the eye
- **Eyelids** - Protect the eye anteriorly
  - **Palpebral fissure** - separates eyelids

- **Lacrimal caruncle** - elevation at medial commissure; contains oil and sweat glands
- **Tarsal plates** - internal supporting connective tissue sheet
- **Levator palpebrae superioris** - gives the upper eyelid mobility
- **Eyelashes** - Nerve endings of follicles initiate reflex blinking
- **Lubricating glands** associated with the eyelids
  - **Tarsal (Meibomian) glands** – Secretion keeps the eyelids from sticking together
  - **Sebaceous glands** associated with follicles
  - **Ciliary glands** between the hair follicles
- **Conjunctiva** - Transparent membrane produces a lubricating mucous secretion
  - **Palpebral conjunctiva** lines the eyelids
  - **Bulbar conjunctiva** covers the white of the eyes
- **Lacrimal Apparatus** - Lacrimal gland and ducts that connect to nasal cavity
  - **Tears**: Dilute saline solution containing mucus, antibodies, and lysozyme
  - Blinking spreads the tears toward the medial commissure; tears enter paired **lacrimal canaliculi** via the **lacrimal puncta**; drain into the **nasolacrimal duct**
- **Extrinsic Eye Muscles** - Six strap-like extrinsic eye muscles that enable the eye to follow moving objects; originate from the bony orbit; maintain the shape of the eyeball
  - Four **rectus muscles** (inferior, superior, lateral, medial): Names indicate the movements they promote
  - Two **oblique muscles** (inferior, superior): Move the eye in the vertical plane and rotate the eyeball laterally (inferior) or medially (superior)

Figure 14.1 Eyeball, cross-section

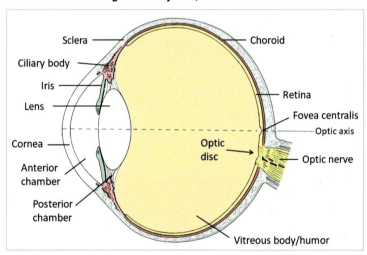

Structure of the Eyeball
- The **wall** of eyeball contains three layers: Fibrous, vascular, sensory
- The **internal cavity** is filled with fluids called **humors**
- The **lens** separates the internal cavity into anterior and posterior segments (cavities)

- **Fibrous Layer** - Outermost layer; dense avascular connective tissue
  - **Sclera** - Opaque posterior region; protects and shapes eyeball; anchors extrinsic

eye muscles
- **Cornea** - Transparent anterior 1/6 of fibrous layer; bends light as it enters the eye; numerous pain receptors contribute to blinking and tearing reflexes
- **Vascular Layer (Uvea)** - Middle pigmented layer
  - **Choroid region** - Posterior portion of the uvea; supplies blood to all layers of the eyeball; brown pigment absorbs light to prevent visual confusion
  - **Ciliary body** - Ring of tissue surrounding the lens; smooth muscle bundles (**ciliary muscles**) control lens shape; capillaries of **ciliary processes** secrete fluid; **ciliary zonule** (suspensory ligament) holds lens in position
  - **Iris** - The colored part of the eye
    - **Pupil** - central opening that regulates the amount of light entering the eye
      - Close vision and bright light - **sphincter papillae** contracts; pupils constrict
      - Distant vision and dim light - **dilator papillae** contracts; pupils dilate
      - Changes in emotional state - pupils dilate when the subject matter is appealing or requires problem-solving skills
- **Sensory Layer**: **Retina** - Delicate two-layered membrane
  - **Pigmented layer** - Outer layer; absorbs light and prevents its scattering; stores vitamin A
  - **Neural layer** - **Photoreceptors**: transduce light energy
    - **Rods** - More numerous at peripheral region of retina, away from the macula lutea
      - Operate in **dim light**; provide **indistinct, fuzzy, non-color peripheral vision**
    - **Cones** - Found in the **macula lutea**; concentrated in the **fovea centralis**
      - Operate in **bright light**; provide **high-acuity color vision**
    - Ganglion cell axons run along the inner surface of the retina
    - Leave the eye as the **optic nerve**
  - **Optic disc** (blind spot) - Site where the optic nerve leaves the eye
    - Lacks photoreceptors

Figure 14.2 Circulation of aqueous humor

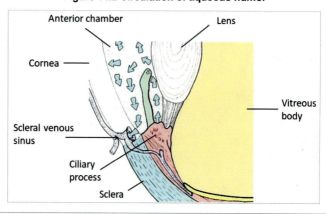

Internal Chambers and Fluids
- The lens and ciliary zonule separate the anterior and posterior segments
  - **Posterior segment** contains **vitreous humor/body** that:

- Transmits light
- Supports the posterior surface of the lens
- Holds the neural retina firmly against the pigmented layer
- Contributes to intraocular pressure
- **Anterior segment** is composed of two chambers
- **Anterior chamber** - between the cornea and the iris
- **Posterior chamber** - between the iris and the lens
- Anterior segment contains **aqueous humor**
- Plasma like fluid continuously filtered from capillaries of the **ciliary processes**
- Drains via the **scleral venous sinus** (canal of Schlemm) at the sclera-cornea junction
- Supplies nutrients and oxygen mainly to the lens and cornea but also to the retina, and removes wastes
- **Glaucoma**: compression of the retina and optic nerve if drainage of aqueous humor is blocked

Lens
- Biconvex, transparent, flexible, elastic, and avascular
- Allows precise focusing of light on the retina
- Cells of **lens epithelium** differentiate into **lens fibers** that form the bulk of the lens
  - **Lens fibers** - cells filled with the transparent protein **crystallin**
- Lens becomes denser, more convex, and less elastic with age
- **Cataracts** (clouding of lens) occur as a consequence of aging, diabetes mellitus, heavy smoking, and frequent exposure to intense sunlight

Physiology of Vision

Light: packets of energy called photons (quanta) that travel in a wavelike fashion
- Our eyes respond to visible light, a small portion of the electromagnetic spectrum
- Rods and cones respond to different wavelengths of the visible spectrum

Refraction: Bending of a light ray due to change in speed when light passes from one transparent medium to another
- Occurs when light meets the surface of a different medium at an oblique angle
- Light passing through a convex lens is bent so that the rays converge at a focal point
- Light is refracted
  - At the cornea
  - Entering the lens
  - Leaving the lens
- Change in lens curvature allows for fine focusing of an image

Focusing for Distant Vision
- Light rays from distant objects are nearly parallel at the eye and need little refraction beyond what occurs in the at-rest eye
- **Far point of vision**: the distance beyond which no change in lens shape is needed for focusing; **20 feet for emmetropic (normal) eye**
- Ciliary muscles are relaxed
- Lens is stretched flat by tension in the ciliary zonule

Focusing for Close Vision

- Light from a close object diverges as it approaches the eye; requires that the eye make active adjustments
  - **Accommodation** - changing the lens shape by ciliary muscles to increase refractory power
  - Near point of vision is determined by the maximum bulge the lens can achieve
  - **Presbyopia** - loss of accommodation over age 50
  - **Constriction** - the accommodation pupillary reflex constricts the pupils to prevent the most divergent light rays from entering the eye
  - **Convergence** - medial rotation of the eyeballs toward the object being viewed

Problems of Refraction
- **Myopia (nearsightedness)** - focal point is in front of the retina, e.g. in a longer than normal eyeball; corrected with a concave lens
- **Hyperopia (farsightedness)** - focal point is behind the retina, e.g. in a shorter than normal eyeball; corrected with a convex lens
- **Astigmatism** - caused by unequal curvatures in different parts of the cornea or lens; corrected with cylindrically ground lenses, corneal implants, or laser procedures

Photoreceptors - Rods and cones
- **Outer segment** of each contains **visual pigments** (photopigments) - molecules that change shape as they absorb light
- **Inner segment** of each joins the cell body
- **Rods** - Very sensitive to dim light; best suited for **night vision** and **peripheral vision**; perceived input is in **gray tones** only; **fuzzy and indistinct images**
- **Cones** - Need bright light for activation; have one of three pigments that furnish a vividly **colored, detailed, high-resolution vision**

- **Excitation of Rods**
  - In the dark visual pigment rhodopsin forms and accumulates
  - When light is absorbed, rhodopsin breaks down
  - Retinal and opsin separate **(bleaching of the pigment)**
- **Excitation of Cones**
  - There are **three types of cones**, named for the colors of light absorbed: **blue, green**, and **red**
  - Intermediate hues are perceived by activation of more than one type of cone at the same time
  - **Color blindness** is due to a congenital lack of one or more of the cone types

- **Light Adaptation** - Occurs when moving from darkness into bright light
  - Large amounts of pigments are broken down instantaneously, producing glare
  - Pupils constrict
  - Dramatic changes in retinal sensitivity: rod function ceases
  - Cones and neurons rapidly adapt
  - Visual acuity improves over 5–10 minutes
- **Dark Adaptation** - Occurs when moving from bright light into darkness
  - Cones stop functioning in low-intensity light
  - Pupils dilate
  - Rhodopsin accumulates in the dark and retinal sensitivity increases within 20–30 minutes

- **Visual Pathway**
  - Axons of retinal ganglion cells form the **optic nerve**
  - **Medial fibers** of the optic nerve **decussate at the optic chiasma**
  - Most fibers of the optic tracts continue to the lateral geniculate body of the **thalamus**
  - The optic radiation fibers connect to the **primary visual cortex** in the occipital lobes
- **Depth Perception**
  - Both eyes view the same image from slightly different angles
  - Depth perception (**three-dimensional vision**) results from cortical fusion of the slightly different images

Sense of Smell

- The organ of smell - **olfactory epithelium** in the roof of the nasal cavity
- **Olfactory receptor cells** - bipolar neurons with radiating olfactory cilia
- Bundles of axons of olfactory receptor cells form the filaments of the **olfactory nerve** (cranial nerve I)
- **Supporting cells** surround and cushion olfactory receptor cells
- **Basal cells** lie at the base of the epithelium

Physiology of Smell

- Dissolved **odorants** bind to receptor proteins in the olfactory cilium membranes
- G protein mechanism is activated, which produces cAMP as a second messenger
- cAMP opens Na^+ and Ca^{2+} channels, causing depolarization of the receptor membrane that then triggers an action potential

Olfactory Pathway

- Olfactory receptor cells synapse with mitral cells in glomeruli of the olfactory bulbs
- Mitral cells amplify, refine, and relay signals along the olfactory tracts to the:
  - Olfactory cortex
  - Hypothalamus, amygdala, and limbic system

Figure 14.3 Olfactory epithelium and olfactory pathway

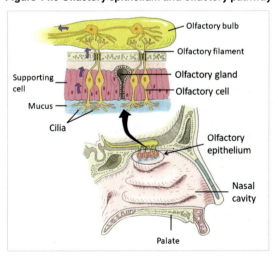

Sense of Taste

- Receptor organs are **taste buds** mostly found on the tongue
  - On the tops of **fungiform papillae**
  - On the side walls of **foliate papillae** and **circumvallate (vallate) papillae**
- Structure of a Taste Bud
  - **Basal cells** - dynamic stem cells
  - **Gustatory cells** - taste cells
  - Microvilli (**gustatory hairs**) project through a taste pore to the surface of the epithelium

Physiology of Taste
- Binding of the food chemical (**tastant**) depolarizes the taste cell membrane, causing release of neurotransmitter that initiates a generator potential that elicits an action potential
- Five basic **taste sensations**
  - **Sweet** - sugars, saccharin, alcohol, and some amino acids
  - **Sour** - hydrogen ions
  - **Salty** - metal ions
  - **Bitter** - alkaloids such as quinine and nicotine
  - **Umami** - amino acids glutamate and aspartate
- **Influence of other sensations on taste**
  - Taste is 80% smell
  - Thermoreceptors, mechanoreceptors, nociceptors in the mouth also influence tastes
  - Temperature and texture enhance or detract from taste

Gustatory Pathway
- **Cranial nerves VII and IX** carry impulses from taste buds to the solitary nucleus of the medulla
- Impulses then travel to the thalamus and from there fibers branch to the:
  - Gustatory cortex in the insula
  - Hypothalamus and limbic system (appreciation of taste)

Figure 14.4 Lingual papillae

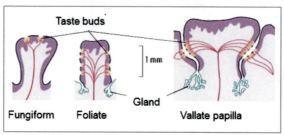

Hearing

- **External ear and middle ear** are involved with **hearing**
- **Internal ear** (labyrinth) functions in both **hearing and equilibrium**
- Receptors for hearing and balance
  - Respond to separate stimuli

- Are activated independently

External Ear
- **Auricle** (pinna) - Composed of **helix** (rim) and **lobul** (earlobe)
- **External acoustic meatus** (auditory canal) - Short, curved tube lined with skin bearing hairs, sebaceous glands, and ceruminous glands
- **Tympanic membrane** (eardrum) - Boundary between external and middle ears; connective tissue membrane that vibrates in response to sound; transfers sound energy to the bones of the middle ear

Middle Ear
- A small, air-filled, mucosa-lined cavity in the temporal bone; flanked medially by bony wall containing the **oval** (vestibular) and **round** (cochlear) **windows**
- **Epitympanic recess** - superior portion of the middle ear
- **Pharyngotympanic (auditory) tube** - connects the middle ear to the nasopharynx; equalizes pressure in the middle ear cavity with the external air pressure
- **Ear Ossicles** - Three small bones in tympanic cavity: **malleus**, **incus**, and **stapes**
  - Suspended by ligaments and joined by synovial joints
  - Transmit vibratory motion of eardrum to oval window

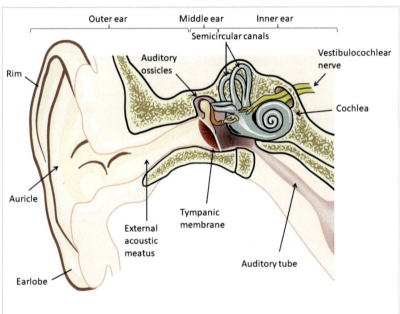

Figure 14.5 Ear, cross-section

Internal Ear
- **Bony labyrinth** - Tortuous channels in the temporal bone filled with **perilymph**
  - Series of **membranous sacs** within the bony labyrinth filled with endolymph
- **Vestibule** - Central egg-shaped cavity of the bony labyrinth
  - **Saccule** is continuous with the cochlear duct
  - **Utricle** is continuous with the semicircular canals

- House equilibrium receptor regions – **maculae**
- **Respond to gravity** and changes in the position of the head
- **Semicircular Canals**
  - **Three canals** (anterior, lateral, and posterior) that each define two-thirds of a circle
  - **Membranous semicircular ducts** line each canal and communicate with the utricle
  - Ampulla of each canal houses equilibrium receptor region called the **crista ampullaris**
  - Receptors respond to **angular (rotational) movements** of the head
- **Cochlea** - Spiral, conical, bony chamber
  - Extends from the vestibule; coils around a bony pillar (**modiolus**)
  - The cavity of the cochlea is divided into three chambers
    - **Scala vestibuli** - abuts the oval window, contains perilymph
    - **Scala media** (cochlear duct) - contains endolymph
    - **Scala tympani** - terminates at the round window; contains perilymph
  - The scalae tympani and vestibuli are continuous with each other at the **helicotrema** (apex)
  - The roof of the cochlear duct is the **vestibular membrane**; the floor is composed of:
    - The bony **spiral lamina**
    - The **basilar membrane**, which supports the **organ of Corti**
  - The **cochlear branch of nerve VIII** runs from the organ of Corti to the brain

Physiology of Hearing

Transmission of Sound to the Internal Ear

Air conduction
- Sound waves vibrate the tympanic membrane → ossicles vibrate and amplify the pressure at the oval window → pressure waves move through perilymph of the scala vestibuli → waves with frequencies below the threshold of hearing travel through the helicotrema and scala tympani to the round window
- Sounds in the hearing range go through the cochlear duct, vibrating the basilar membrane at a specific location, according to the frequency of the sound
- Fibers that span the width of the basilar membrane are short and stiff near oval window, and resonate in response to high-frequency pressure waves.
- Longer fibers near the apex resonate with lower-frequency pressure waves

Bone conduction
- Sound is transmitted to the bones of the skull
- Bones are denser than air and, thus, conduct lower frequencies
- We perceive our own voices to be lower and fuller than others do

- Cells of the **spiral organ**
  - **Supporting cells**
  - **Cochlear hair cells**
- **Stereocilia** protrude into the endolymph; enmeshed in the gel-like tectorial membrane
- Bending stereocilia opens mechanically gated ion channels, inward K^+ and Ca^{2+} current causes a graded potential and the release of neurotransmitter glutamate
- **Cochlear fibers** transmit impulses to the **auditory cortex** via the thalamus
- Auditory pathways decussate so that both cortices receive input from both ears

Homeostatic Imbalances of Hearing
- **Conduction deafness** - Blocked sound conduction to the fluids of the internal ear
  - Can result from impacted earwax, perforated eardrum, or otosclerosis of the ossicles
- **Sensorineural deafness** - Damage to the neural structures at any point from the cochlear hair cells to the auditory cortical cells

Figure 14.6 Air conduction of sound

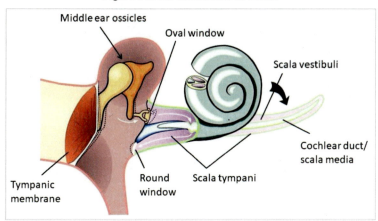

Balance and Equilibrium

- Vestibular apparatus consists of:
  - **Vestibular receptors** that monitor **static equilibrium**
  - **Semicircular canal receptors** that monitor **dynamic equilibrium**

Maculae - Sensory receptors for static equilibrium
- One in each saccule wall and one in each utricle wall; monitor the position of the head in space, necessary for control of posture
- **Respond to linear acceleration** forces, but not rotation
- Stereocilia and kinocilia are embedded in the **otolithic membrane** studded with **otoliths** (tiny $CaCO_3$ stones)
- Bending of hairs in the direction of the kinocilia or the opposite direction increases or reduces the rate of impulse generation → informs brain of changing position of head

Crista Ampullaris (Crista) - Sensory receptor for dynamic equilibrium
- Major stimuli are rotatory movements
- One in the ampulla of each semicircular canal; each crista has hair cells that extend into a gel-like mass called the cupula
- Cristae respond to changes in velocity of rotatory movements of the head
- Bending of hairs in the cristae causes rapid impulses or fewer impulses reach the brain → informs brain of rotational movements of the head

Equilibrium Pathway to the Brain
- Pathways are complex; impulses travel to the vestibular nuclei in the brain stem or the cerebellum, both of which receive other input
- Three modes of input for balance and orientation
  - Vestibular receptors

- Visual receptors
- Somatic receptors

Figure 14.7 Inner ear with receptors for static and dynamic equilibrium

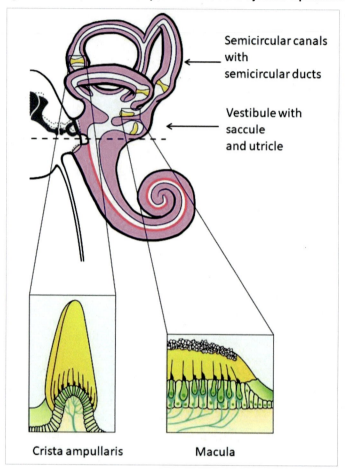

A&P Essentials 4th ed.

Chapter 15 Endocrine System

Endocrine glands: pituitary, thyroid, parathyroid, adrenal, and pineal glands
- Some organs produce both hormones and exocrine products (e.g., pancreas and gonads)
- The **hypothalamus** has both neural and endocrine functions
- Other tissues and organs that produce hormones include adipose cells, thymus, cells in the walls of the small intestine, stomach, kidneys, and heart

- **Hormones**: long-distance chemical signals that travel in the blood or lymph
- **Autocrines**: chemicals that exert effects on the same cells that secrete them
- **Paracrines**: locally acting chemicals that affect other cells
  - **Amino acid-based hormones** - Amines, thyroxine, peptides, and proteins
  - **Steroids** - Synthesized from cholesterol; gonadal and adrenocortical hormones
  - **Mechanisms of Hormone Action**
  - **Water-soluble hormones** (all amino acid–based hormones **except thyroid hormone**) - Cannot enter the target cells; act on plasma membrane receptors → coupled by G proteins to intracellular second messengers that mediate the target cell's response
  - **Lipid-soluble hormones** (steroid and thyroid hormones) - Act on intracellular receptors that directly activate genes

Target Cell Specificity - Target cells must have specific receptors to which the hormone binds
Target cell activation depends on:
- Blood levels of the hormone
- Relative number of receptors on or in the target cell
- Affinity of binding between receptor and hormone
- Hormones influence the number of their receptors
  - **Up-regulation** - target cells form more receptors in response to the hormone
  - **Down-regulation** - target cells lose receptors in response to the hormone

Hormones circulate **in the blood** either free or bound
- **Steroids and thyroid hormone** are attached to **plasma proteins**
- All others circulate without carriers
- The concentration of a circulating hormone reflects:
  - Rate of release
  - Speed of inactivation and removal from the body
- Hormones are removed from the blood by
  - Degrading enzymes
  - Kidneys
  - Liver
- **Half-life** - the time required for a hormone's blood level to decrease by half

Interaction of Hormones at Target Cells
- **Permissiveness**: one hormone cannot exert its effects without another hormone being present
- **Synergism**: more than one hormone produces the same effects on a target cell
- **Antagonism**: one or more hormones opposes the action of another hormone

Control of Hormone Release
- Blood levels of hormones are controlled by negative feedback systems; vary only within a narrow desirable range
- Hormones are synthesized and released in response to stimuli:
  - **Humoral Stimuli**: Changing blood levels of ions and nutrients directly stimulates secretion of hormones; e.g., Ca^{2+} in the blood
  - **Neural Stimuli**: Nerve fibers stimulate hormone release; e.g., sympathetic nervous system fibers stimulate the adrenal medulla to secrete catecholamines
  - **Hormonal Stimuli**: Hormones stimulate other endocrine organs to release their hormones; e.g., hypothalamic hormones stimulate the release of most anterior pituitary hormones
- **Hypothalamic-pituitary-target endocrine organ feedback loop**: hormones from the final target organs inhibit the release of the

Nervous System Modulation
- The nervous system modifies the stimulation of endocrine glands and their negative feedback mechanisms; e.g., under severe stress, the hypothalamus and the sympathetic nervous system are activated → body glucose levels rise

Figure 15.1 Major endocrine glands

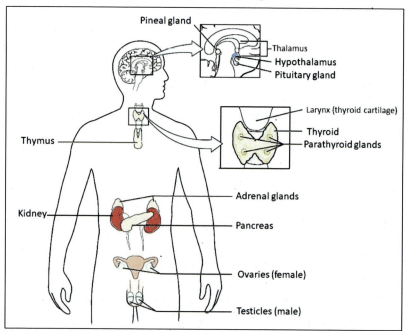

Endocrine glands/tissues and hormones

Pituitary gland (hypophysis) has two major lobes
- **Posterior pituitary** (neurohypophysis): Downgrowth of hypothalamic neural tissue
  - Nuclei of the hypothalamus synthesize the neurohormones **oxytocin** and **antidiuretic hormone** (ADH); transported to the posterior pituitary via **hypothalamic-hypophyseal tract**

- **Anterior pituitary** (adenohypophysis): Glandular tissue; originates as an outpocketing of the oral mucosa
- **Hypophyseal portal system**: Carries **releasing** and **inhibiting hormones** to the anterior pituitary to regulate hormone secretion
- **Anterior Pituitary Hormones** are proteins; TSH, ACTH, FSH, and LH are all tropic hormones (regulate the secretory action of other endocrine glands)

Figure 15.2 Hypothalamus-anterior pituitary-target organ axis

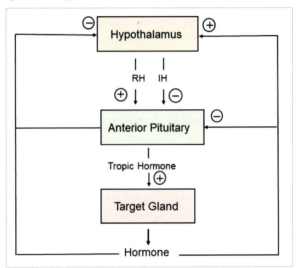

Growth Hormone (GH)	• Stimulates most cells, but targets bone and skeletal muscle
	• Promotes protein synthesis and encourages use of fats for fuel
	• Most effects are mediated indirectly by **insulin-like growth factors** (IGFs)
	• **GH release** is regulated by
	  • **Growth hormone–releasing hormone** (GHRH)
	  • **Growth hormone–inhibiting hormone** (GHIH) (somatostatin)
	• **Hypersecretion**: In children → **gigantism**, in adults → **acromegaly**
	• **Hyposecretion**: In children → pituitary dwarfism

Thyroid-Stimulating Hormone (TSH, Thyrotropin)	• Stimulates the normal development and secretory activity of the thyroid
	• **Regulation of TSH release**
	  • Stimulated by **thyrotropin-releasing hormone** (TRH)
	  • Inhibited by rising blood levels of thyroid hormones that act on the pituitary and hypothalamus

Adrenocorticotropic Hormone (ACTH, Corticotropin)	• Stimulates the adrenal cortex to release corticosteroids • **Regulation of ACTH release** • Triggered by hypothalamic **corticotropin-releasing hor-**

	mone (CRH) in a **daily rhythm** • Internal and external factors such as fever, hypoglycemia, and stressors can alter the release of CRH

Gonadotropins	• **Follicle-stimulating hormone (FSH)** stimulates gamete (egg or sperm) production
	• **Luteinizing hormone (LH)** promotes production of **gonadal hormones**
	• Absent from the blood in prepubertal boys and girls
	• **Regulation of gonadotropin release**
	  • Triggered by the **gonadotropin-releasing hormone (GnRH)** during and after puberty
	  • Suppressed by gonadal hormones (feedback)

Prolactin (PRL)	• Stimulates **milk production** • Regulation of PRL release • Primarily controlled by prolactin-inhibiting hormone (PIH) (**dopamine**) • Blood levels rise toward the end of pregnancy • Suckling stimulates PRH release and promotes continued milk production
Posterior Pituitary Hormones are released in response to nerve impulses	
Oxytocin	• Stimulates uterine contractions during childbirth by mobilizing Ca^{2+} • Also triggers **milk ejection** ("letdown" reflex) in women producing milk • Plays a role in **sexual arousal and orgasm** in both sexes

Antidiuretic Hormone (ADH)	• Hypothalamic osmoreceptors respond to changes in the solute concentration of the blood
	  • If solute concentration is high ADH is synthesized and released, inhibiting urine formation
	  • If solute concentration is low ADH is not released, allowing water loss
	• **Alcohol** inhibits ADH release and causes copious urine output

Thyroid Gland
• Consists of **two** lateral **lobes** connected by a median mass called the **isthmus**
• Composed of **follicles** that produce the glycoprotein **thyroglobulin**
• Colloid (thyroglobulin + iodine) fills the lumen of the follicles and is the precursor of **thyroid hormone**
• **Parafollicular cells** produce the hormone **calcitonin**

	• Major metabolic hormone; increases metabolic rate and heat production (calorigenic effect); plays a role in
	  • Maintenance of blood pressure
	  • Regulation of tissue growth
	  • Development of skeletal and nervous systems
	  • Reproductive capabilities

Thyroid Hormone (TH)	• T_4 **(thyroxine)** & T_3 **(triiodothyronine)** are transported by **thyroxine-binding globulins** (TBGs)
	• T_3 **is ten times more active than** T_4; peripheral tissues convert T_4 to T_3
	• **Negative feedback regulation** of TH release
	  • Rising TH levels provide negative feedback inhibition on release of TSH
	  • **Hypothalamic thyrotropin-releasing hormone** (TRH) can overcome the negative feedback during pregnancy or exposure to cold
	• **Hyposecretion in adults** - myxedema; endemic goiter if due to lack of iodine
	• **Hyposecretion in infants** - cretinism
	• **Hypersecretion** - Graves' disease

Calcitonin	• Produced by **parafollicular (C) cells** • Antagonist to parathyroid hormone (PTH) • Inhibits osteoclast activity and release of Ca^{2+} from bone matrix • Stimulates Ca^{2+} uptake and incorporation into bone matrix • Regulated by a humoral (Ca^{2+} concentration in the blood) negative feedback mechanism • No important role in humans; removal of thyroid (and its C cells) does not affect Ca^{2+} homeostasis

Parathyroid glands
• Four to eight tiny glands embedded in the posterior aspect of the thyroid
• **Chief cells** secrete **parathyroid hormone**
• PTH - most important hormone in Ca^{2+} homeostasis

Parathyroid Hormone (PTH, parathormone)	• Stimulates osteoclasts to digest bone matrix
	• Enhances reabsorption of Ca^{2+} and secretion of phosphate by the kidneys
	• Promotes activation of vitamin D (by the kidneys); increases absorption of Ca^{2+} by intestinal mucosa
	• **Negative feedback control**: rising Ca^{2+} in the blood inhibits PTH release
	• **Hyperparathyroidism** due to tumor
	  • Bones soften and deform
	  • Elevated Ca^{2+} depresses the nervous system and contributes to formation of kidney stones
	• **Hypoparathyroidism** following gland trauma or removal results in tetany, respiratory paralysis, and death

Adrenal (Suprarenal) Glands
• Paired, pyramid-shaped organs atop the kidneys
• **Adrenal medulla** - nervous tissue; part of the sympathetic nervous system
  • Chromaffin cells secrete **epinephrine** (80%) and **norepinephrine** (20%)
  • These hormones cause blood glucose levels to rise, blood vessels to constrict, the heart to beat faster, blood to be diverted to the brain, heart, and skeletal muscle

- **Epinephrine** stimulates metabolic activities, bronchial dilation, and blood flow to skeletal muscles and the heart
- **Norepinephrine** influences peripheral vasoconstriction and blood pressure
- **Adrenal cortex** - three layers of glandular tissue that synthesize and secrete corticosteroids
  - **Zona glomerulosa** - mineralocorticoids
  - **Zona fasciculata** - glucocorticoids
  - **Zona reticularis** - sex hormones or gonadocorticoids

Mineralocorticoids	• Regulate electrolytes (primarily Na^+ and K^+) in ECF
	• **Aldosterone**, the **most potent mineralocorticoid**, stimulates Na^+ reabsorption and water retention by the kidneys
	• Mechanisms of Aldosterone Secretion
	  • **Renin-angiotensin mechanism**: Decreased blood pressure stimulates kidneys to release renin, triggers formation of angiotensin II, a potent stimulator of aldosterone release
	  • **Plasma concentration of K+**: Increased K+ directly influences the zona glomerulosa cells to release aldosterone
	  • **ACTH**: causes small increases of aldosterone during stress

Glucocorticoids	• Keep blood sugar levels relatively constant • Maintain blood pressure by increasing the action of vasoconstrictors • **Cortisol** is the **most significant glucocorticoid** • Released in response to ACTH, patterns of eating and activity, and stress • **Prime metabolic effect is gluconeogenesis** - formation of glucose from fats and proteins • Promotes rises in blood glucose, fatty acids, and amino acids

Gonadocorticoids (Sex Hormones)	• Most are **androgens** that are converted to testosterone in tissue cells or estrogens in females
	• May contribute to
	  • The onset of puberty
	  • The appearance of secondary sex characteristics
	  • Sex drive

Pineal Gland
- Small gland hanging from the roof of the third ventricle
- Pinealocytes secrete melatonin, derived from serotonin
- **Melatonin**
  - Timing of sexual maturation and puberty
  - Day/night cycles
  - Physiological processes that show rhythmic variations (body temperature, sleep, appetite)

Pancreas
- Has both exocrine and endocrine cells

- Acinar cells (**exocrine**) produce an **enzyme-rich juice** for digestion
- **Pancreatic islets** (islets of Langerhans) contain **endocrine cells**
  - **Alpha (α) cells** produce glucagon
  - **Beta (β) cells** produce insulin

Glucagon	• Major target is the liver, where it promotes • **Glycogenolysis** - breakdown of glycogen to glucose • **Gluconeogenesis** - synthesis of glucose from lactic acid and noncarbohydrates • Release of glucose to the blood
Insulin	• Lowers blood glucose levels • Enhances membrane transport of glucose into fat and muscle cells • Participates in neuronal development and learning and memory • Inhibits glycogenolysis and gluconeogenesis

Ovaries and Placenta
- Gonads produce steroid **sex hormones**
- **Ovaries** produce **estrogens and progesterone** responsible for:
  - Maturation of female reproductive organs
  - Appearance of female secondary sexual characteristics
  - Breast development and cyclic changes in the uterine mucosa
- The **placenta** secretes **estrogens**, **progesterone**, and **human chorionic gonadotropin** (hCG)
- The **testes** produce **testosterone** that
  - Initiates maturation of male reproductive organs
  - Causes appearance of male secondary sexual characteristics and sex drive
  - Is necessary for normal sperm production
  - Maintains reproductive organs in their functional state

Other Hormone-Producing Tissues/Organs

Heart	• **Atrial natriuretic peptide** (ANP) reduces blood pressure, blood volume, and blood Na^+ concentration
Gastrointestinal tract (Enteroendocrine cells)	• **Gastrin** stimulates release of HCl • **Secretin** stimulates liver and pancreas • **Cholecystokinin** stimulates pancreas, gallbladder, and hepatopancreatic sphincter
Kidneys	• **Erythropoietin** regulates production of red blood cells • **Renin** initiates the renin-angiotensin mechanism
Skin	• **Cholecalciferol**, the precursor of vitamin D
Adipose tissue	• **Leptin** is involved in appetite control, and stimulates increased energy expenditure • Secreted by fat cells in response to increased body fat mass • Indicator of total energy stores in fat tissue

	• Important for timing of puberty
Skeleton (osteoblasts)	• **Osteocalcin** prods pancreatic beta cells to divide and secrete more insulin, improving glucose handling and reducing body fat
Thymus	• **Thymulin, thymopoietins**, and **thymosins** are involved in normal development of the T lymphocytes in the immune response

Chapter 16 Cardiac Anatomy & Physiology

Anatomy

- Approximately the size of a fist
- Located in the mediastinum between second rib and fifth intercostal space; on the superior surface of diaphragm; 2/3 to the left of the midsternal line; anterior to the vertebral column, posterior to the sternum
- Apex points toward left hip

Pericardium

- **Superficial fibrous pericardium:** Protects, anchors, and prevents overfilling
- Deep two-layered **serous pericardium**
  - **Parietal layer** lines the internal surface of the fibrous pericardium
  - **Visceral layer (epicardium)** on external surface of the heart
  - Separated by fluid-filled **pericardial cavity** (decreases friction)

Layers of the Heart Wall

- **Epicardium** - Visceral layer of the serous pericardium
- **Myocardium** - Spiral bundles of cardiac muscle cells
  - **Fibrous skeleton of the heart**: crisscrossing, interlacing layer of connective tissue; anchors cardiac muscle fibers; supports great vessels and valves; limits spread of action potentials to specific paths
- **Endocardium** is continuous with endothelial lining of blood vessels

Figure 16.1 Heart, anterior view

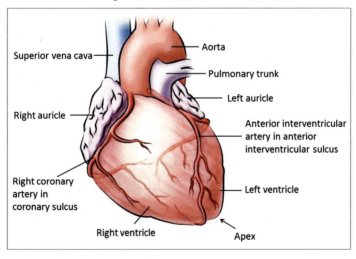

Chambers
- **Atria**: Receiving Chambers
  - Separated internally by the **interatrial septum**
  - **Coronary sulcus** (atrioventricular groove) encircles the junction of atria and ventricles
  - **Auricles** increase atrial volume

- Walls are ridged by **pectinate muscles**
- **Vessels entering right atrium:** Superior vena cava, inferior vena cava, coronary sinus
- **Vessels entering left atrium:** Right and left pulmonary veins
- **Ventricles**: Discharging Chambers
  - Separated by the **interventricular septum**
  - **Anterior and posterior interventricular sulci** mark the position of the septum externally
  - Walls are ridged by **trabeculae carneae**
  - **Papillary muscles** project into the ventricular cavities
  - **Vessel leaving the right ventricle** - Pulmonary trunk
  - **Vessel leaving the left ventricle** - Aorta

Figure 16.2 Heart, cross-section

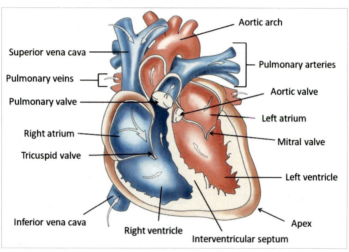

Heart Valves - Ensure unidirectional blood flow through the heart
- **Atrioventricular (AV) valves** - Prevent backflow into the atria when ventricles contract
  - **Tricuspid valve** – between right atrium and ventricle
  - **Mitral (bicuspid) valve** – between left atrium and ventricle
  - **Chordae tendineae** anchor AV valve cusps to papillary muscles
- **Semilunar (SL) valves** - Prevent backflow into the ventricles when ventricles relax
  - **Aortic (semilunar) valve** – between left ventricle and aorta
  - **Pulmonary (semilunar) valve** – between right ventricle and pulmonary trunk

Pathway of Blood Through the Heart
- The heart is **two side-by-side pumps**
- **Right side** is the pump for the **pulmonary circuit** - short, low-pressure circulation that carries blood to and from the lungs
- **Left side** is the pump for the **systemic circuit** - long pathways that carries blood to and from all body tissues
- Right atrium → tricuspid valve → right ventricle → pulmonary valve → pulmonary

trunk → pulmonary arteries → lungs → pulmonary veins → left atrium → bicuspid valve → left ventricle → aortic valve → aorta → systemic circulation
- Equal volumes of blood are pumped to the pulmonary and systemic circuits

Coronary Circulation - The functional blood supply to the heart muscle itself
- Arterial supply varies considerably and contains many anastomoses (junctions) among branches
- Collateral routes provide additional routes for blood delivery
- **Arteries:** Right and left coronary (in atrioventricular groove), marginal, circumflex, and anterior and posterior interventricular arteries
- **Veins:** Small cardiac, anterior cardiac, and great cardiac veins

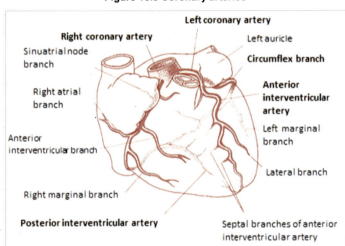

Figure 16.3 Coronary arteries

Cardiac Muscle Cells

- Cardiac muscle cells are striated, short, fat, branched, and interconnected
- Connective tissue matrix (**endomysium**) connects to the fibrous skeleton
- **T tubules** are wide but less numerous; **SR** is simpler than in skeletal muscle
- Numerous large mitochondria (25–35% of cell volume)
- **Intercalated discs**: junctions between cells anchor cardiac cells
  - Desmosomes prevent cells from separating during contraction
- **Gap junctions** allow ions to pass; electrically couple adjacent cells
- **Heart muscle behaves as a functional syncytium**

Cardiac Physiology

Cardiac Muscle Contraction
- **Depolarization of the heart is rhythmic and spontaneous**
- About 1% of cardiac cells have automaticity - (are self-excitable)
- **Gap junctions** ensure the heart contracts as a unit
- **Long absolute refractory period** (250 ms)
- Depolarization opens voltage-gated fast Na^+ channels → reversal of membrane poten-

tial from –90 mV to +30 mV → depolarization wave in T tubules causes the SR to release Ca^{2+} and opens slow **Ca^{2+} channels** in the sarcolemma
- Ca^{2+} surge prolongs the depolarization phase (**plateau**)
- Ca^{2+} influx triggers opening of Ca^{2+}-sensitive channels in the SR, which liberates bursts of Ca^{2+}
- E-C coupling occurs as Ca^{2+} binds to troponin and sliding of the filaments begins
- **Duration of the AP** and the contractile phase is **much greater** in cardiac muscle **than in skeletal muscle**
- Repolarization results from inactivation of Ca^{2+} channels and opening of voltage-gated K^+ channels

Cardiac Conduction System

Intrinsic cardiac conduction system
- A network of noncontractile (autorhythmic) cells that initiate and distribute impulses to coordinate the depolarization and contraction of the heart
- **Autorhythmic Cells** - Have unstable resting potentials (pacemaker potentials) due to open slow Na^+ channels
  - At threshold, Ca^{2+} channels open → explosive Ca^{2+} influx produces the rising phase of the action potential
  - Repolarization results from inactivation of Ca^{2+} channels and opening of voltage-gated K^+ channel

Figure 16.4 Intrinsic conduction system

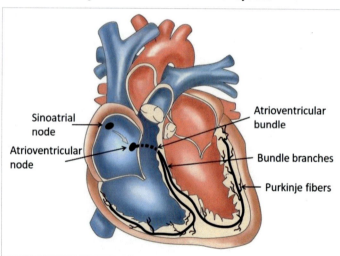

Sequence of Excitation
- **Sinoatrial (SA) node** (pacemaker) - Generates impulses about 90-95 times/minute **(sinus rhythm)**; depolarizes faster than any other part of the myocardium
- **Atrioventricular (AV) node** - Smaller diameter fibers; fewer gap junctions; delays impulses approximately 0.1 second; Depolarizes 40-60 times per minute in absence of SA node input
- **Atrioventricular (AV) bundle (bundle of His)** - Only electrical connection between

the atria and ventricles
- **Right and left bundle branches** - Two pathways in the interventricular septum that carry the impulses toward the apex of the heart
- **Purkinje fibers** - Complete the pathway into the apex and ventricular walls
- AV bundle and Purkinje fibers depolarize only 30-40 times per minute in absence of AV node input

Defects in the intrinsic conduction system may result in
- **Arrhythmia**: Irregular heart rhythm - Uncoordinated atrial and ventricular contractions
- **Fibrillation**: Rapid, irregular contractions; useless for pumping blood
- **Defective SA node** may result in **ectopic focus**; abnormal pacemaker takes over
  - If AV node takes over, there will be a **junctional rhythm** (40–60 bpm)
- **Defective AV node** may result in **partial or total heart block** - few or no impulses from SA node reach the ventricles

Extrinsic Innervation of the Heart
- Heartbeat is modified by the ANS
- **Cardiac centers** are located in the medulla oblongata
  - **Cardioacceleratory center** innervates SA and AV nodes, heart muscle, and coronary arteries through sympathetic neurons
  - **Cardioinhibitory center** inhibits SA and AV nodes through parasympathetic fibers in the vagus nerves

- **Electrocardiogram** (ECG or EKG): a composite of all the action potentials generated by nodal and contractile cells at a given time
- Three waves
  - **P wave**: depolarization of SA node
  - **QRS complex**: ventricular depolarization
  - **T wave**: ventricular repolarization

Figure 16.5 Standard ECG

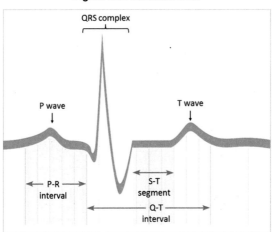

Heart Sounds

- Two sounds (lub-dup) **associated with closing of heart valves**

A&P Essentials 4th ed.

- **First sound** occurs as AV valves close and signifies beginning of systole
- **Second sound** occurs when SL valves close at the beginning of ventricular diastole
- **Heart murmurs**: abnormal heart sounds most often indicative of valve problems

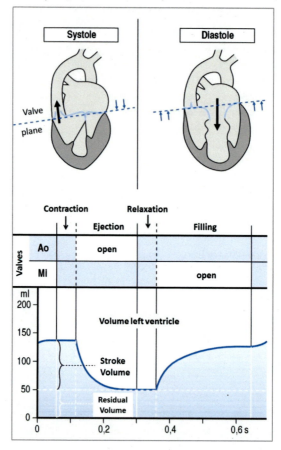

Figure 16.6 Cardiac cycle left ventricle

Cardiac cycle

All events associated with blood flow through the heart during one complete heartbeat
- **Systole** - contraction
- **Diastole** - relaxation
- **Phases of the Cardiac Cycle**
  - **Ventricular filling** - takes place in mid-to-late diastole
    - AV valves are open
    - 80% of blood passively flows into ventricles
    - **Atrial systole** occurs, delivering the remaining 20%
    - **End-diastolic volume** (EDV): volume of blood in each ventricle at the end of ventricular diastole

- **Ventricular systole**
  - Atria relax and ventricles begin to contract
  - Rising ventricular pressure results in closing of AV valves
  - **Isovolumetric contraction** phase (all valves are closed)
  - In **ejection phase**, ventricular pressure exceeds pressure in the large arteries, forcing the SL valves open
  - **End-systolic volume** (ESV): volume of blood remaining in each ventricle
  - **Isovolumetric relaxation** occurs in early diastole
  - Ventricles relax
  - Backflow of blood in aorta and pulmonary trunk closes SL valves and causes **dicrotic notch** (brief dip in aortic pressure)

Cardiac Output

Volume of blood pumped by each ventricle in one minute
- CO = heart rate (HR) x stroke volume (SV)
  - HR = number of beats per minute
  - SV = volume of blood pumped out by a ventricle with each beat = EDV - ESV
- At rest - CO (ml/min) = HR (75 beats/min) $\times$ SV (70 ml/beat) = **5.25 l/min**
- **Maximal CO** is 4–5 times resting CO in nonathletic people; may reach 35 l/min in trained athletes
- **Cardiac reserve**: difference between resting and maximal CO

Regulation of Stroke Volume
- **Preload**: degree of stretch of cardiac muscle cells before they contract (**Frank-Starling law of heart**)
  - Cardiac muscle exhibits a length-tension relationship → at rest, cardiac muscle cells are shorter than optimal length
  - Slow heartbeat and exercise increase venous return → distends (stretches) the ventricles and increases contraction force
- **Contractility**: contractile strength at a given muscle length, independent of muscle stretch and EDV
  - **Positive inotropic agents** increase contractility; e.g., increased Ca^{2+} influx due to sympathetic stimulation, hormones (thyroxine, glucagon, and epinephrine)
  - **Negative inotropic agents** decrease contractility, e.g., Ca^{2+} channel blockers
- **Afterload**: pressure that must be overcome for ventricles to eject blood
  - Hypertension increases afterload, resulting in increased ESV and reduced SV

Regulation of Heart Rate
- **Positive chronotropic factors** increase heart rate
- **Negative chronotropic factors** decrease heart rate
- **Autonomic Nervous System Regulation**
  - **Sympathetic nervous system** is activated by emotional or physical stressors
    - Norepinephrine causes the pacemaker to fire more rapidly (and at the same time increases contractility)
  - **Parasympathetic nervous system** opposes sympathetic effects
    - Acetylcholine hyperpolarizes pacemaker cells by opening K^+ channels
    - The heart at rest exhibits vagal tone (parasympathetic)
  - **Atrial (Bainbridge) reflex**: a sympathetic reflex initiated by increased venous return

- Stretch of the atrial walls stimulates the SA node
- Also stimulates atrial stretch receptors activating sympathetic reflexes

Chemical Regulation of Heart Rate
- **Hormones**
  - Epinephrine from adrenal medulla enhances heart rate and contractility
  - Thyroxine increases heart rate and enhances the effects of norepinephrine and epinephrine
  - **Intra- and extracellular ion concentrations** (e.g., Ca^{2+} and K^+) must be maintained for normal heart function

A&P Essentials 4th ed.

Chapter 17 Blood Vessels & Circulation

Blood Vessel Anatomy

* Delivery system of dynamic structures that begins and ends at the heart
  * **Arteries**: carry blood away from the heart; oxygenated except for pulmonary circulation and umbilical vessels of a fetus
  * **Capillaries**: contact tissue cells and directly serve cellular needs
  * **Veins**: carry blood toward the heart
* **Structure of Blood Vessel Walls**
  * **Arteries and veins** - Tunica intima, tunica media, and tunica externa
  * **Capillaries** - Endothelium with sparse basal lamina

* **Tunica intima** - Endothelium lines the lumen of all vessels
  * In vessels larger than 1 mm, a subendothelial connective tissue basement membrane is present
* **Tunica media** - Smooth muscle and sheets of elastin
  * Sympathetic vasomotor nerve fibers control vasoconstriction and vasodilation of vessels
* **Tunica externa** (tunica adventitia) - Collagen fibers protect and reinforce
  * Larger vessels contain vasa vasorum to nourish the external layer

Elastic (Conducting) Arteries - Large thick-walled arteries with elastin in all three tunics
* **Aorta and its major branches**
  * Large lumen offers low-resistance
  * Act as pressure reservoirs - expand and recoil as blood is ejected from the heart

Muscular (Distributing) Arteries and Arterioles - Distal to elastic arteries; deliver blood to organs
* Thick tunica media with more smooth muscle
* Active in vasoconstriction

Arterioles - Smallest arteries
* **Control flow into capillary beds** via vasodilation and vasoconstriction

Capillaries - Microscopic blood vessels
* Walls of thin tunica intima, one cell thick
* **Pericytes** help stabilize their walls and control permeability
* Size allows only a single RBC to pass at a time
* In all tissues except for cartilage, epithelia, cornea and lens of eye
* *Functions*: exchange of gases, nutrients, wastes, hormones, etc.
* **Continuous Capillaries** - Abundant in the skin and muscles
  * Tight junctions connect endothelial cells
  * Intercellular clefts allow the passage of fluids and small solutes
* **Fenestrated Capillaries** - Some endothelial cells contain pores (fenestrations)
  * More permeable than continuous capillaries
  * Function in absorption or filtrate formation)
* **Sinusoidal Capillaries** - Fewer tight junctions, larger intercellular clefts, large lumens
  * Usually fenestrated

- Allow large molecules and blood cells to pass between the blood and surrounding tissues
- Found in the liver, bone marrow, spleen

Venules - Formed when capillary beds unite
- Very porous; allow fluids and WBCs into tissues
- Postcapillary venules consist of endothelium and a few pericytes
- Larger venules have one or two layers of smooth muscle cells

Veins - Formed when venules converge
- Have thinner walls, larger lumens compared with corresponding arteries as blood pressure is lower than in arteries
- Thin tunica media and a thick tunica externa consisting of collagen fibers and elastic networks
- Called **capacitance vessels** (blood reservoirs); contain up to 65% of the blood supply
- Adaptations that ensure return of blood to the heart
  - Large-diameter lumens offer little resistance
  - Valves prevent backflow of blood
- Most abundant in veins of the limbs
- **Venous sinuses**: flattened veins with extremely thin walls (e.g., coronary sinus of the heart and dural sinuses of the brain)

Vascular Anastomoses - Interconnections of blood vessels
- **Arterial anastomoses** provide alternate pathways (collateral channels) to a given body region; common at joints, in abdominal organs, brain, and heart
- Vascular shunts of capillaries are examples of **arteriovenous anastomoses**
- **Venous anastomoses** are common

Blood pressure

Blood flow - Volume of blood flowing through a vessel, an organ, or the entire circulation in a given period
- Equivalent to cardiac output (CO) for entire vascular system
- Relatively constant when at rest
- Varies widely through individual organs, based on needs

Blood pressure (BP) - Force exerted on the wall of a blood vessel by the blood
- Expressed in mm Hg
- **Measured as systemic arterial BP in large arteries near the heart**
- The pressure gradient provides the driving force that keeps blood moving from higher to lower pressure areas

Resistance (peripheral resistance) - Opposition to flow
- Measure of the amount of friction blood encounters
- Generally encountered in the peripheral systemic circulation
- Three important sources of resistance
  - **Blood viscosity** - The "stickiness" of the blood due to formed elements and plasma proteins
  - **Blood vessel length** - The longer the vessel, the greater the resistance
  - **Blood vessel diameter** - Frequent changes alter **peripheral resistance**

- Varies inversely with the fourth power of vessel radius, e. g., if the radius is doubled, the resistance is 1/16 as much
- **Small-diameter arterioles are the major determinants of peripheral resistance**

Systemic Blood Pressure
- Is highest in the aorta
- Declines throughout the pathway
- Is 0 mm Hg in the right atrium
- **Arterial Blood Pressure** reflects two factors of the arteries close to the heart
- **Elasticity** (compliance or distensibility)
- **Volume of blood** forced into them at any time
- Blood pressure near the heart is pulsatile
- **Systolic pressure**: pressure exerted during ventricular contraction
- **Diastolic pressure**: lowest level of arterial pressure
- **Pulse pressure** = difference between systolic and diastolic pressure
- **Mean arterial pressure** (MAP): pressure that propels the blood to the tissues
- MAP = diastolic pressure + 1/3 pulse pressure
- **Capillary Blood Pressure** - Ranges from 15 to 35 mm Hg
- High BP would rupture fragile, thin-walled capillaries
- Most are very permeable, so low pressure forces filtrate into interstitial spaces
- **Venous Blood Pressure**
- Changes little during the cardiac cycle
- Small pressure gradient, about 15 mm Hg
- Low pressure due to cumulative effects of peripheral resistance

Factors Aiding Venous Return
- **Respiratory "pump"**: pressure changes created during breathing move blood toward the heart by squeezing abdominal veins as thoracic veins expand
- **Muscular "pump"**: contraction of skeletal muscles "milk" blood toward the heart and valves prevent backflow
- **Vasoconstriction** of veins under sympathetic control

Figure 17.1 Capillary bed

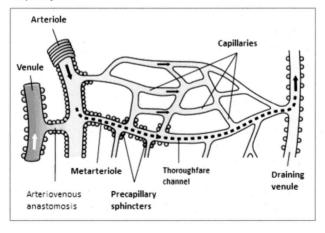

Table 17.1 Blood Pressure Classification for Adults

Category	Systolic BP (mm Hg)		Diastolic BP (mm Hg)
Normal blood pressure	< 120	and	< 80
Elevated blood pressure (prehypertension)	120-129	and	< 80
Stage 1 hypertension	130-139	or	80-89
Stage 2 hypertension	≥ 160	or	≥ 90

Maintenance and control of blood pressure

Maintaining Blood Pressure requires
- Cooperation of the heart, blood vessels, and kidneys
- Supervision by the brain
- The **main factors influencing blood pressure**:
  - Cardiac output (CO)
  - Peripheral resistance (PR)
  - Blood volume
- **Blood pressure varies directly with CO, PR, and blood volume**
- Changes in one variable are quickly compensated for by changes in the other variables

Control of Blood Pressure
- **Short-term neural and hormonal controls** - Counteract fluctuations in blood pressure by altering peripheral resistance
- **Long-term renal regulation** - Counteracts fluctuations in blood pressure by altering blood volume

Neural controls of peripheral resistance
- Maintain MAP by altering blood vessel diameter
- Alter blood distribution in response to specific demands
- Operate via reflex arcs that involve
  - Baroreceptors
  - Vasomotor centers and vasomotor fibers
  - Vascular smooth muscle
- **Vasomotor Center** - A cluster of sympathetic neurons in the medulla that oversee changes in blood vessel diameter
  - Maintains vasomotor tone (moderate constriction of arterioles)
  - Receives inputs from baroreceptors, chemoreceptors, and higher brain center
- **Baroreceptor-Initiated Reflexes**
  - Baroreceptors are located in the
    - Carotid sinuses
    - Aortic arch
    - Walls of large arteries of the neck and thorax
  - Baroreceptors taking part in the **carotid sinus reflex protect the blood supply to the brain**
  - Baroreceptors taking part in the **aortic reflex** help maintain adequate blood pressure in the **systemic circuit**

- **Chemoreceptor-Initiated Reflexes** - More important in the regulation of respiratory rate (see **Chapter 20: Respiratory System**)
- **Influence of Higher Brain Centers**
  - Reflexes that regulate BP are integrated in the medulla
  - Higher brain centers (cortex and hypothalamus) can modify BP via relays to medullary centers

Hormonal Controls
- Adrenal medulla hormones **norepinephrine** (NE) and **epinephrine** cause generalized vasoconstriction and increase cardiac output
- **Angiotensin II**, generated by kidney release of renin, causes vasoconstriction
- **Atrial natriuretic peptide** causes blood volume and blood pressure to decline, causes generalized vasodilation
- **Antidiuretic hormone** (ADH, vasopressin) causes intense vasoconstriction in cases of extremely low BP

Renal Regulation
- **Direct Mechanism** - Alters blood volume independently of hormones
  - **Increased BP** or blood volume causes the kidneys to eliminate more urine, thus reducing BP
  - **Decreased BP** or blood volume causes the kidneys to conserve water, and BP rises
- **Indirect Mechanism - Renin-angiotensin mechanism**
  - ↓ Arterial blood pressure → release of renin → production of angiotensin II → aldosterone secretion
  - **Aldosterone** → renal reabsorption of Na^+ and ↓ urine formation
  - Angiotensin II stimulates **ADH** release

Figure 17.2 Baroreceptor-initiated regulation of systemic blood pressure

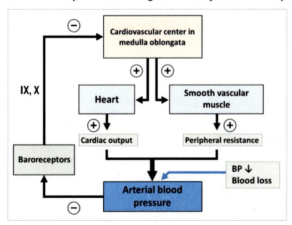

Vital signs: pulse and blood pressure, along with respiratory rate and body temperature

Measuring Systemic arterial BP
- Measured indirectly by the auscultatory method using a sphygmomanometer
- Pressure is released slowly and the examiner listens for **sounds of Korotkoff** with a stethoscope

- Sounds first occur as blood starts to spurt through the artery (**systolic pressure**, normally **110–140 mm Hg**)
- Sounds disappear when the artery is no longer constricted and blood is flowing freely (**diastolic pressure**, normally **70–80 mm Hg**)

Variations in Blood Pressure
- Blood pressure cycles over a 24-hour period
- BP peaks in the morning due to levels of hormones
- Age, sex, weight, race, mood, and posture may vary BP

Blood Flow through Organs and Tissues

Tissue Perfusion
- Is involved in
  - Delivery of O_2 and nutrients to, and removal of wastes from, tissue cells
  - Gas exchange (lungs)
  - Absorption of nutrients (digestive tract)
  - Urine formation (kidneys)
- Rate of flow is precisely the right amount to provide for proper function
- **Velocity of Blood Flow** - Changes as it travels through the systemic circulation
  - Is fastest in the aorta, slowest in the capillaries, increases again in veins
    - Slow capillary flow allows adequate time for exchange between blood and tissues

Autoregulation - Automatic adjustment of blood flow to each tissue in proportion to its requirements at any given point in time
- Is controlled intrinsically by modifying the diameter of local arterioles feeding the capillaries
- Is independent of MAP, which is controlled as needed to maintain constant pressure
- **Metabolic Controls** - Vasodilation of arterioles and relaxation of precapillary sphincters occur in response to
  - Declining tissue O_2
  - Substances from metabolically active tissues (H^+, K^+, adenosine, prostaglandins) and inflammatory chemicals
  - Leads to relaxation of vascular smooth muscle
  - Release of NO from vascular endothelial cells
    - **NO** is the **major factor causing vasodilation**
  - **Vasoconstriction** is due to sympathetic stimulation and endothelins
- **Myogenic Controls** - Myogenic responses of vascular smooth muscle keep tissue perfusion constant despite most fluctuations in systemic pressure
  - Passive stretch (increased intravascular pressure) promotes increased tone and vasoconstriction
  - Reduced stretch promotes vasodilation and increases blood flow to the tissue

Long-Term Autoregulation
- **Angiogenesis** - The number of vessels to a region increases and existing vessels enlarge; common in the heart when a coronary vessel is occluded

Perfusion of organs/organ systems	
Skeletal Mus-	• At **rest**, myogenic and general neural mechanisms predominate

cles	• During **muscle activity** blood flow increases in direct proportion to the metabolic activity (active or exercise hyperemia) • Local controls override sympathetic vasoconstriction • Muscle blood flow can increase 10× or more during physical activity

Brain	• **Blood flow to the brain is constant**, as neurons are intolerant of ischemia
	• **Metabolic controls**: Declines in pH, and increased carbon dioxide cause marked vasodilation
	• **Myogenic controls**
	  • Decreases in MAP cause cerebral vessels to dilate
	  • Increases in MAP cause cerebral vessels to constrict
	  • The brain is vulnerable under extreme systemic pressure changes
	  • MAP below 60 mm Hg can cause syncope (fainting)
	  • MAP above 160 can result in cerebral edema

Skin	• Blood flow to venous plexuses below the skin surface varies from 50 ml/min to 2500 ml/min, depending on body temperature
	• Is controlled by sympathetic nervous system reflexes initiated by temperature receptors and the central nervous system
	• As **temperature rises** (e.g., heat exposure, fever, vigorous exercise)
	  • Hypothalamic signals reduce vasomotor stimulation of the skin vessels
	  • Heat radiates from the skin
	  • Sweat also causes vasodilation via bradykinin in perspiration
	  • Bradykinin stimulates the release of NO
	• As **temperature decreases**, blood is shunted to deeper, more vital organs

Lungs	• Arteries/arterioles are thin walled with large lumens • Arterial resistance and pressure are low (24/8 mm Hg) • Autoregulatory mechanism is opposite of that in most tissues • Low O_2 levels cause vasoconstriction; high levels promote vasodilation • Allows for proper O_2 loading in the lungs

Heart	• During **ventricular systole** coronary vessels are compressed
	  • Myocardial blood flow ceases
	  • Stored myoglobin supplies sufficient oxygen
	• At **rest**, control is probably myogenic
	• During **strenuous exercise** coronary vessels dilate in response to local accumulation of vasodilators
	  • Blood flow may increase three to four times

Microcirculation

Capillary Exchange
• Diffusion of

- O_2 and nutrients from the blood to tissues
- CO_2 and metabolic wastes from tissues to the blood
- **Lipid-soluble molecules** diffuse directly through endothelial membranes
- **Water-soluble solutes** pass through clefts and fenestrations
- **Larger molecules**, such as proteins, are **actively transported**

Bulk Flow
- Extremely important in determining relative fluid volumes in the blood and interstitial space
- Direction and amount of fluid flow depends on two opposing forces: hydrostatic and colloid osmotic pressures
  - **Hydrostatic Pressures**
    - **Capillary hydrostatic pressure** (= capillary blood pressure) forces fluids through the capillary walls; is greater at the arterial end of a bed than at the venule end
    - **Interstitial fluid hydrostatic pressure** assumed to be zero because of lymphatic vessels
  - **Colloid Osmotic Pressures**
    - **Capillary colloid osmotic pressure** (= oncotic pressure) created by plasma proteins, which draw water toward themselves
    - **Interstitial fluid osmotic pressure** low (~1 mm Hg) due to low protein content
- **Net Filtration Pressure (NFP)** - comprises all the forces acting on a capillary bed
  - At the **arterial end** of a bed, hydrostatic forces dominate → **fluid leaves the capillary**
  - At the **venous end**, osmotic forces dominate → **fluid moves back into the vessel**
- Excess fluid is returned to the blood via the lymphatic system

Figure 17.3 Frank-Starling Law of Bulk flow

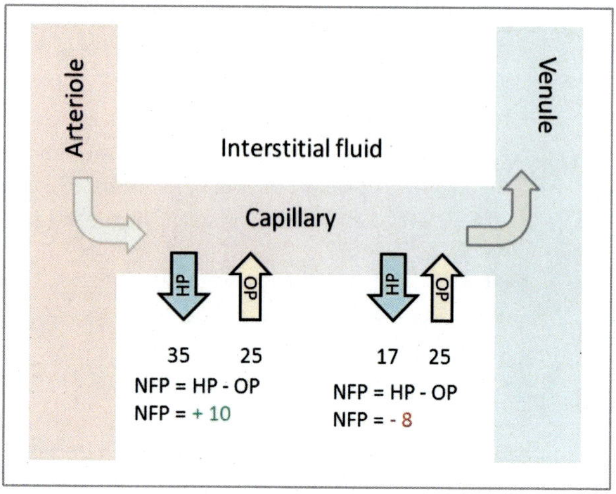

Arteriole | Venule
Interstitial fluid
Capillary

35 25
NFP = HP - OP
NFP = + 10

17 25
NFP = HP - OP
NFP = - 8

Circulatory Pathways

- Two main circulations
- **Pulmonary circulation**: short loop that runs from the heart to the lungs and back to the heart

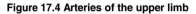

- **Systemic circulation**: long loop to all parts of the body and back to the heart

Figure 17.4 Arteries of the upper limb

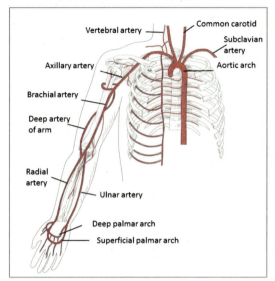

Major Arteries of the Systemic Circulation

Artery	Description
Coronary arteries	• Branch off of the aorta just behind the aortic valve. • Supply the myocardium of ventricles and atria. • Major branches are **right and left coronary arteries, marginal artery, circumflex artery, anterior and posterior interventricular arteries**.
Brachiocephalic trunk	• First branch of the aortic arc. • Splits into right common carotid artery and right subclavian artery.
Common carotid artery	• Branches off of the brachiocephalic trunk (right side) and the aortic arch (left side). • Splits into external and internal carotid arteries.
External carotid artery	• Branches off of the common carotid arteries. • Supplies most of the head, but not the brain.
Internal carotid artery	• Branches off of the common carotid arteries. • Supplies 80% of the brain.
Subclavian artery	• Branches off the brachiocephalic trunk (right side) and the aortic arch (left side). • Supplies the tissue of the upper limb. • Changes its name to **axillary artery** when entering the axilla, and to **brachial artery** once it emerges from the axilla. • Splits just below the elbow into its two end branches:

	the **radial artery** on the lateral side and the **ulnar artery** on the medial side of the arm. • The **radial artery** is rather superficial at the root of the thumb, which makes this spot the most commonly used site for pulse palpation.
Vertebral artery	• Branches off of the subclavian artery. • Ascends and enters the skull through the foramen magnum. Supplies 20% of the brain, including the cerebellum.

Figure 17.5 Arteries of the head

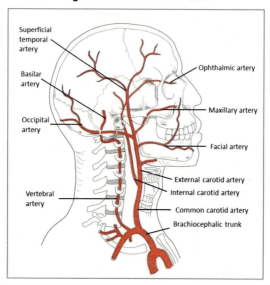

Celiac trunk	• First branch of the abdominal aorta just below the diaphragm. • Splits almost immediately into three branches: **common hepatic artery** (for the liver), **splenic artery** (for the spleen), and **left gastric artery** (for the stomach).
Superior mesenteric artery	• Second branch of the abdominal aorta. • Supplies the pancreas, small intestine and part of the large intestine.
Inferior mesenteric artery	• Third branch of the abdominal aorta. • Supplies the second part of the large intestine.
Renal artery	• Branches off of the abdominal artery and supplies the kidney.
Common iliac artery	• Splits into the **right** and **left common iliac arteries** that supply **the lower limbs** (via the **femoral artery**) and **pelvic organs**.
External iliac artery	• Branches off of the common iliac artery. • Called **femoral artery** once it has passed under the

inguinal ligament and called **popliteal artery** one it reaches the knee area.

- Splits into the **anterior tibial artery** for the anterior part of the leg and the **posterior tibial artery** for the posterior part.

Figure 17.6 Abdominal aorta and major branches

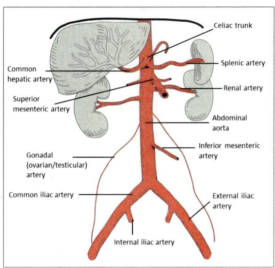

Figure 17.7 Arteries of the lower limb

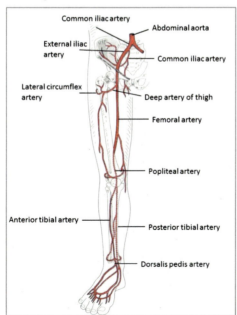

Major Veins of the Systemic Circulation

Vein	Description
Inferior vena cava	• Collects blood from all organs and tissues located below the diaphragm. • Empties into the right atrium.
Superior vena cava	• Collects blood from all organs and tissues located above the diaphragm. • Empties into the right atrium.
Coronary sinus	• Collects the blood from the cardiac tissue. • Empties into the right atrium.
Subclavian vein	• Collects blood from the head (via **external jugular vein** and **vertebral vein**) and upper limb (veins of the upper limb).
Internal jugular vein	• Collects blood from the head (**facial vein, ophthalmic veins**) and brain (**dural venous sinuses**).

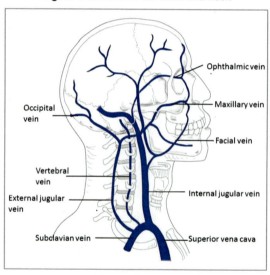

Figure 17.8 Veins of the head and neck

Brachiocephalic vein	• Formed by fusion of **subclavian vein** and **internal jugular vein**.
Azygos vein	• Drains blood from the abdominal and thoracic wall via the **hemiazygos vein** and **accessory hemiazygos vein**.
Veins of upper limb	• The forearm has five main veins called **radial, ulnar, basilic, cephalic**, and **median antebrachial vein**. • The radial and ulnar veins unite to form the **brachial vein** of the arm. • The **median cubital vein** connects basilica and cephalic veins on the anterior side of the elbow.

- The three veins of the arm unite to form the **subclavian vein**.

Figure 17.9 Veins of the upper limb

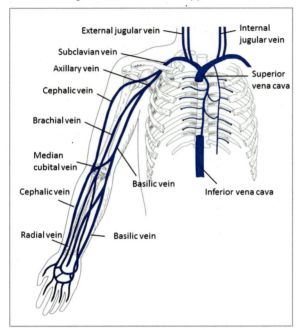

Figure 17.10 Veins of the abdominal cavity

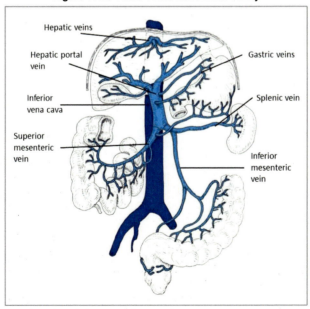

A&P Essentials 4th ed.

Veins of lower limb	• The **lower leg** has two main deep veins (**anterior** and **posterior tibial veins**) and two superficial veins (**small** and **great saphenous veins**). • The deep veins and the small saphenous vein form the **popliteal vein**, which is called **femoral vein** above the popliteal fossa. • Once **inside the pelvis**, the femoral vein is called the **external iliac vein**. • It unites with the **internal iliac vein** to form the **common iliac vein**, and the two common iliac veins join to form the **inferior vena cava**.

Figure 17.11 Veins of the lower limb

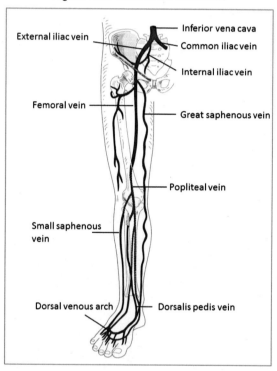

146

A&P Essentials 4th ed.

Chapter 18 Blood, Hemostasis, and Blood Groups

Blood Composition

Blood: a fluid connective tissue composed of
- Plasma
- Formed elements

Hematocrit - Percent of blood volume that is RBCs
- 47% ± 5% for males
- 42% ± 5% for females

[handwritten: anemia - red is low; polycythemia - red is high]

Physical Characteristics and Volume
- Sticky, opaque fluid
- Color scarlet to dark red
- pH 7.35–7.45
- 100.4° F (38°C)
- ~8% of body weight
- Average volume: 5–6 l for males, and 4–5 l for females

Hematopoiesis (hemopoiesis): Blood cell formation occurs in red bone marrow of axial skeleton, girdles and proximal epiphyses of humerus and femur
- **Hemocytoblasts** (hematopoietic stem cells) - Give rise to all formed elements
- Hormones and growth factors push the cell toward a specific pathway of blood cell development
- New blood cells enter blood sinusoids

Figure 18.1 Formation of formed blood elements in the bone marrow

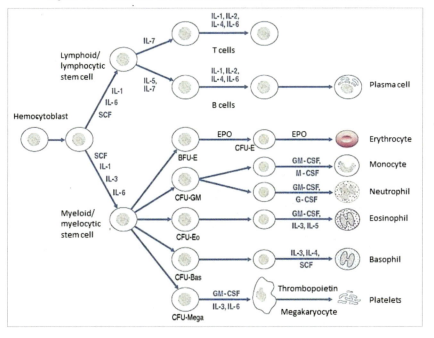

Plasma
- 90% **water**
- **Proteins** are mostly produced by the liver
  - 60% albumin
  - 36% globulins
  - 4% fibrinogen
- **Nitrogenous by-products of metabolism** - lactic acid, urea, creatinine
- **Nutrients** - glucose, carbohydrates, amino acids
- **Electrolytes** - Na^+, K^+, Ca^{2+}, Cl^-, HCO_3^-
- **Respiratory gases** - O_2 and CO_2
- **Hormones**

Formed Elements
- Only WBCs are complete cells
- RBCs have no nuclei or organelles
- Platelets are cell fragments
- Most formed elements survive in the bloodstream for only a few days
- Most blood cells originate in bone marrow and do not divide

Figure 18.2 Blood cells (formed elements)

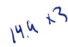

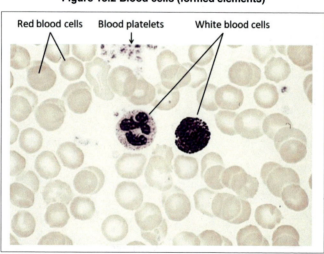

Erythrocytes

- Biconcave discs, anucleate, essentially no organelles
- Filled with hemoglobin (Hb) for gas transport
- Are the major factor contributing to blood viscosity
- Structural characteristics contribute to gas transport
- Biconcave shape - huge surface area relative to volume
- >97% hemoglobin (not counting water)
- No mitochondria; ATP production is anaerobic; no O_2 is used in generation of ATP

RBCs are dedicated to respiratory gas transport

- Hemoglobin binds reversibly with oxygen
- Hemoglobin structure
  - Protein **globin**: two alpha and two beta chains
  - **Heme** pigment bonded to each globin chain
  - **Iron** atom in each heme can bind to one O_2 molecule
- Each Hb molecule can transport four O_2
- O_2 **loading** in the lungs - Produces **oxyhemoglobin** (ruby red)
- O_2 **unloading** in the tissues - Produces **deoxyhemoglobin** or reduced hemoglobin (dark red)
- CO_2 loading in the tissues - Produces **carbaminohemoglobin** (carries 20% of CO_2 in the blood)

Erythropoiesis - Red blood cell production
- Hemocytoblast → proerythroblast → erythroblast → reticulocyte (released into blood) → mature erythrocyte

Regulation of Erythropoiesis
- Hormonal controls
- Adequate supplies of iron, amino acids, and B vitamins

- **Hormonal Control**
  - **Erythropoietin (EPO)**
    - Direct stimulus for erythropoiesis
    - Released by the kidneys (10% liver) in response to hypoxia
      - **Causes of hypoxia**
        - Hemorrhage or increased RBC destruction reduces RBC numbers
        - Insufficient hemoglobin (e.g., iron deficiency)
        - Reduced availability of O_2 (e.g., high altitudes)
      - **Effects of EPO**
        - More rapid maturation of committed bone marrow cells
        - Increased circulating reticulocyte count in 1–2 days
  - **Testosterone** also enhances EPO production, resulting in higher RBC counts in males
- **Dietary Requirements** for Erythropoiesis
  - **Nutrients** - amino acids, lipids, and carbohydrates
  - **Iron** - Stored in Hb (65%), the liver, spleen, and bone marrow
    - Stored in cells as ferritin and hemosiderin
    - Transported loosely bound to the protein transferrin
  - **Vitamin B_{12} and folic acid** - necessary for DNA synthesis for cell division

Fate and Destruction of Erythrocytes
- **Life span**: 100–120 days
- Old RBCs become fragile, and Hb begins to degenerate → macrophages engulf old RBCs in the spleen and liver → heme and globin separated
  - Iron salvaged for reuse
  - Heme degraded to yellow bilirubin → liver secretes bilirubin (in bile) into the intestines
  - Degraded pigment leaves the body in feces as stercobilin
  - Globin is metabolized into amino acids

A&P Essentials 4th ed.

Leukocytes 4,500 - 11,000

- Make up <1% of total blood volume
- Can leave capillaries via diapedesis
- Move through tissue spaces by ameboid motion and positive chemotaxis
- **Leukocytosis**: WBC count over 11,000/mm$_3$
  - Normal response to bacterial or viral invasion

- **Granulocytes**
  - Neutrophils, eosinophils, and basophils
  - Cytoplasmic granules stain specifically with Wright's stain
  - Lobed nuclei
  - Phagocytic

Neutrophils	• Most numerous WBCs • **Polymorphonuclear leukocytes** (PMNs) • Fine granules take up both acidic and basic dyes; give cytoplasm a lilac color • Granules contain hydrolytic enzymes or defensins • Very phagocytic - "bacteria slayers"
Eosinophils	• Red-staining, bilobed nuclei • Red to crimson (acidophilic) coarse, lysosome-like granules • Digest parasitic worms that are too large to be phagocytized • Modulators of the immune response
Basophils	• Rarest WBCs • Large, purplish-black (basophilic) granules contain histamine • **Histamine**: an inflammatory chemical that acts as a vasodilator and attracts other WBCs to inflamed sites

Agranulocytes
- Lack visible cytoplasmic granules
- Have spherical or kidney-shaped nuclei

Lymphocytes
mature in bone marrow
	• Large, dark-purple, circular nuclei with a thin rim of blue cytoplasm
	• Mostly in lymphoid tissue; few circulate in the blood
	• Crucial to immunity
	• Two types — *thymus*
	  • **T cells** act against virus-infected cells and tumor cells
	  • **B cells** give rise to plasma cells, which produce antibodies

Monocytes	• The largest leukocytes • Abundant pale-blue cytoplasm • Dark purple-staining, U- or kidney-shaped nuclei • Leave circulation, enter tissues, and **differentiate into macrophages** • Actively phagocytic cells; crucial against viruses, intracellular bacterial parasites, and chronic infections • Activate lymphocytes to mount an immune response

Leukopoiesis
- Production of WBCs is stimulated by chemical messengers from bone marrow and mature WBCs
  - Interleukins (e.g., IL-1, IL-2)
  - Colony-stimulating factors (CSFs) named for the WBC type they stimulate (e.g., granulocyte-CSF stimulates granulocytes)
- All leukocytes originate from hemocytoblasts

Platelets
- Small fragments of **megakaryocytes**
- Formation is regulated by **thrombopoietin**
- Blue-staining outer region, purple granules
- Granules contain serotonin, Ca^{2+}, enzymes, ADP, and platelet-derived growth factor (PDGF)
- Form a temporary platelet plug that helps seal breaks in blood vessels
- Circulating platelets are kept inactive and mobile by NO and prostacyclin from endothelial cells of blood vessels

Normal Values for Blood and Blood Elements

Blood volume	8% of body weight; 5-6 l for men and 4-5 l for women
Color	bright red (oxygen-rich blood) to dark red (oxygen-depleted blood)
pH	7.35 – 7.45
Plasma	55% of total blood volume; 3 l for men and 2.5 l for women
Red blood cell (RBC) count	4.7 – 6.1 million/µL blood male 4.2 – 5.4 million/µL blood female
Hematocrit (HCT)	47% (42 – 52%) male 42% (37 – 47%) female
Hemoglobin (Hb)	16 (14 – 18) g/100 mL blood male 14 (12 – 16) g/100 mL blood female
White blood cell (WBC) count	4,800 – 10,800/µL blood
Neutrophils	3,000 – 7,000/µL blood (50 – 70% of WBC)
Lymphocytes	1,500 – 3,000/µL blood (25 – 40% of WBC)
Monocytes	150 – 800/µL blood (3 – 8% of WBC)
Eosinophils	100 – 400/µL blood (2 – 4% of WBC)
Basophils	20 – 50/µL blood (0.5 – 1% of WBC)
Platelet count	140,000 – 450,000/µL blood

Hemostasis
- Fast series of reactions for stoppage of bleeding
  - Vascular spasm

- Platelet plug formation
- Coagulation (blood clotting)

Vascular Spasm - Vasoconstriction of damaged blood vessel
- Triggered by:
  - Direct injury
  - Chemicals released by endothelial cells and platelets
  - Pain reflexes

Platelet Plug Formation
- Positive feedback cycle
  - At site of blood vessel injury, platelets
  - Stick to exposed collagen fibers with the help of von Willebrand factor, a plasma protein
  - Swell, become spiked and sticky, and release chemical messengers
  - ADP causes more platelets to stick and release their contents
  - Serotonin and thromboxane A_2 enhance vascular spasm and more platelet aggregation

Coagulation - A set of reactions in which blood is transformed from a liquid to a gel
- Reinforces the platelet plug with fibrin threads
- Three phases of coagulation
  - **Prothrombin activator** is formed (intrinsic and extrinsic pathways)
  - Prothrombin is converted into **thrombin**
  - Thrombin catalyzes the joining of fibrinogen to form a **fibrin mesh**
- **Coagulation Phase 1: Two Pathways to Prothrombin Activator**
  - Initiated by either the **intrinsic** or **extrinsic pathway** (usually both)
  - Each pathway cascades toward factor X that complexes with Ca^{2+}, PF_3, and factor V to form prothrombin activator
  - **Intrinsic pathway** - Triggered by negatively charged surfaces (activated platelets, collagen, glass); uses factors present within the blood (intrinsic)
  - **Extrinsic pathway** - Triggered by exposure to tissue factor (TF) or factor III (an extrinsic factor); bypasses several steps of the intrinsic pathway, so is faster
- **Coagulation Phase 2: Pathway to Thrombin**
  - Prothrombin activator catalyzes the transformation of prothrombin to the active enzyme thrombin
- **Coagulation Phase 3: Common Pathway to the Fibrin Mesh**
  - Thrombin converts soluble fibrinogen into fibrin
  - Thrombin (with Ca^{2+}) activates factor XIII which:
    - Cross-links fibrin
    - Strengthens and stabilizes the clot
- **Clot Retraction**
  - Actin and myosin in platelets contract within 30–60 minutes
  - Platelets pull on the fibrin strands, squeezing serum from the clot
- **Factors Limiting Clot Growth or Formation**
  - Swift removal and dilution of clotting factors
  - Inhibition of activated clotting factors

Clot Repair

- **Platelet-derived growth factor** (PDGF) stimulates division of smooth muscle cells and fibroblasts to rebuild blood vessel wall
- **Vascular endothelial growth factor** (VEGF) stimulates endothelial cells to multiply and restore the endothelial lining

Fibrinolysis
- Begins within two days
- Plasminogen in clot is converted to plasmin by **tissue plasminogen activator** (tPA), factor XII and thrombin
- **Plasmin** is a fibrin-digesting enzyme

Inhibition of Clotting Factors
- Most thrombin is bound to fibrin threads, and prevented from acting elsewhere
- Antithrombin III, protein C, and heparin inactivate thrombin and other procoagulants
- Heparin, another anticoagulant, also inhibits thrombin activity

Factors Preventing Undesirable Clotting
- Platelet adhesion is prevented by
  - Smooth endothelial lining of blood vessels
  - Antithrombic substances nitric oxide and prostacyclin secreted by endothelial cells
  - Vitamin E quinine, which acts as a potent anticoagulant

Human Blood Groups

- RBC membranes bear 30 types glycoprotein antigens that are
  - Perceived as foreign if transfused blood is mismatched
  - Unique to each individual
  - Promoters of agglutination and are called agglutinogens
- Presence or absence of each antigen is used to classify blood cells into different groups
- Antigens of the **ABO** and **Rh blood groups** cause vigorous transfusion reactions
- **Other blood groups** (MNS, Duffy, Kell, and Lewis) are usually weak agglutinogens

ABO Blood Groups	• Types A, B, AB, and O based on the presence or absence of two agglutinogens (A and B) on the surface of the RBCs • Blood may contain anti-A or anti-B antibodies (agglutinins) that act against transfused RBCs with ABO antigens not normally present • Anti-A or anti-B form in the blood at about 2 months of age
Rh Blood Groups	• There are 45 different Rh agglutinogens (Rh factors); C, D, and E are most common • Rh$^+$ indicates presence of D • Anti-Rh antibodies are not spontaneously formed in Rh$^-$ individuals • Anti-Rh antibodies form if an Rh$^-$ individual receives Rh$^+$ blood • A second exposure to Rh$^+$ blood will result in a typical transfusion reaction

Hemolytic Disease of the Newborn (also called erythroblastosis fetalis)
- Rh$^-$ mother becomes sensitized when exposure to Rh$^+$ blood causes her body to synthesize anti-Rh antibodies
- Anti-Rh antibodies cross the placenta and destroy the RBCs of an Rh$^+$ baby
- The baby can be treated with prebirth transfusions and exchange transfusions after

birth
- RhoGAM serum containing anti-Rh can prevent the Rh– mother from becoming sensitized

Blood Typing ABO blood groups
- When serum containing anti-A or anti-B agglutinins is added to blood, agglutination will occur between the agglutinin and the corresponding agglutinogens
- Positive reactions indicate agglutination

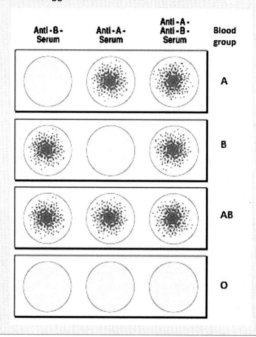

Transfusions
- **Whole-blood transfusions** are used when blood loss is substantial
- **Packed red cells** (plasma removed) are used to restore oxygen-carrying capacity
- **Transfusion Reactions occur if mismatched blood is infused**
  - Donor's cells
    - Are attacked by the recipient's plasma agglutinins
    - Agglutinate and clog small vessels
    - Rupture and release free hemoglobin into the bloodstream
  - Results in
    - Diminished oxygen-carrying capacity
    - Hemoglobin in kidney tubules and renal failure

A&P Essentials 4th ed.

Chapter 19 Lymphatic System and Immunity

Lymphatic System
- Consists of three parts
  - Lymphatic vessels (lymphatics)
  - Lymph
  - Lymph nodes
- Returns interstitial fluid and leaked plasma proteins back to the blood
- Once interstitial fluid enters lymphatics, it is called **lymph**
- On average 3 l of lymph are transported each; can increase up to 20x if necessary
- Together with lymphoid organs and tissues, provide the structural basis of the immune system

Lymphatic Vessels - One-way system, lymph flows toward the heart
- **Lymphatic Capillaries**
  - Similar to blood capillaries, except
    - Very permeable (take up cell debris, pathogens, and cancer cells)
    - Endothelial cells overlap to form one-way minivalves, and are anchored by collagen filaments, preventing collapse of capillaries
    - Absent from bones, teeth, bone marrow and the CNS
  - **Lacteals**: specialized lymph capillaries present in intestinal mucosa absorb digested fat and deliver fatty lymph (**chyle**) to the blood
- **Lymphatic Collecting Vessels**
  - Similar to veins, except
    - Have thinner walls, with more internal valves
    - Anastomose more frequently
- **Lymphatic trunks and ducts**
  - Lymph is delivered into one of two large ducts
    - **Right lymphatic duct** drains the right upper arm and the right side of the head and thorax
    - **Thoracic duct** arises from the cisterna chyli and drains the rest of the body
  - Each empties lymph into venous circulation at the junction of the internal jugular and subclavian veins on its own side of the body

Lymph Transport
- Lymph is propelled by
  - Pulsations of nearby arteries
  - Contractions of smooth muscle in the walls of the lymphatics

Lymphoid Cells

- **Lymphocytes** are the main cells of the immune system; protect against antigens
  - Anything the body perceives as foreign
  - Bacteria and their toxins; viruses
  - Mismatched RBCs or cancer cells
  - **T cells (T lymphocytes)** - Manage the immune response; attack and destroy foreign cells
  - **B cells (B lymphocytes)** - Produce plasma cells, which secrete antibodies

155

A&P Essentials 4th ed.

- **Macrophages** phagocytize foreign substances and help activate T cells
- **Dendritic cells** capture antigens and deliver them to lymph nodes
- **Reticular cells** produce stroma that supports other cells in lymphoid organs

Lymphoid Tissue and Organs

Lymphoid Tissue
- Houses and provides a proliferation site for lymphocytes
- Furnishes a surveillance vantage point
- **Diffuse lymphatic tissue** comprises scattered reticular tissue elements in every body organ
  - Larger collections in the lamina propria of mucous membranes and lymphoid organs
- **Lymphatic follicles** are solid, spherical bodies of tightly packed reticular elements and cells
  - Germinal center composed of dendritic and B cells
  - May form part of larger lymphoid organs

Figure 19.1 Lymph node, cross-section

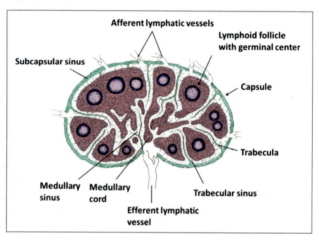

Lymph Nodes
- Embedded in connective tissue, in clusters along lymphatic vessels
- Near the body surface in **inguinal**, **axillary**, and **cervical** regions of the body
- **Filter lymph** - macrophages destroy microorganisms and debris
- **Immune system** - lymphocytes are activated and mount an attack against antigens
- **Structure of a Lymph Node**
  - Bean-shaped
  - External **fibrous capsule**
  - **Trabeculae** extend inward and divide the node into compartments
  - **Cortex** - Contains **follicles** with **germinal centers**, heavy with dividing B cells
    - Dendritic cells nearly encapsulate the follicles
    - Deep cortex houses T cells in transit
    - T cells circulate continuously among the blood, lymph nodes, and lymphatic

stream
- **Medulla** - **Medullary cords** extend inward from the cortex and contain B cells, T cells, and plasma cells
  - **Lymph sinuses** contain macrophages
- **Circulation in the Lymph Nodes**
  - Lymph enters via **afferent lymphatic vessels**
  - Travels through large **subcapsular sinus** and smaller sinuses
  - Exits the node at the hilus via **efferent vessels]**
  - Fewer efferent vessels, causing flow of lymph to stagnate, allowing lymphocytes and macrophages time to carry out functions

Figure 19.2 Spleen, cross-section

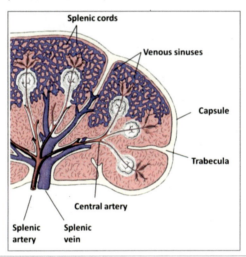

Spleen
- Largest lymphoid organ
- Served by splenic artery and vein, which enter and exit at the hilus
- **Functions**
  - Site of lymphocyte proliferation and immune surveillance and response
  - Cleanses the blood of aged cells and platelets and debris
  - Stores breakdown products of RBCs (e.g., iron) for later reuse
  - Stores blood platelets
  - Site of fetal erythrocyte production (normally ceases after birth)
- Has a **fibrous capsule** and **trabeculae**
- Two distinct areas
  - **White pulp** around central arteries - Mostly lymphocytes on reticular fibers and involved in immune functions
  - **Red pulp** in venous sinuses and splenic cords - Rich in macrophages for disposal of worn-out RBCs and bloodborne pathogens

Thymus
- In infants, it is found in the inferior neck and extends into the mediastinum, where it partially overlies the heart

- Increases in size and is most active during childhood
- Stops growing during adolescence and then gradually atrophies
- **Thymic lobes** contain an outer cortex and inner medulla
- **Cortex** contains densely packed lymphocytes and scattered macrophages
- **Medulla** contains fewer lymphocytes and thymic (Hassall's) corpuscles involved in regulatory T cell development
- Thymus differs from other lymphoid organs in important ways
  - It functions strictly in T lymphocyte maturation
  - It does not directly fight antigens
  - The stroma of the thymus consists of star-shaped epithelial cells (not reticular fibers)
  - These **thymocytes** provide the environment in which T lymphocytes become immunocompetent

Figure 19.3 Tonsil

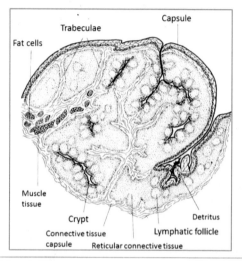

Tonsils - Simplest lymphoid organs
- Form a ring of lymphatic tissue around the pharynx
  - **Palatine tonsils** - at posterior end of the oral cavity
  - **Lingual tonsils** - grouped at the base of the tongue
  - **Pharyngeal tonsil** - in posterior wall of the nasopharynx
  - **Tubal tonsils** - surrounding the openings of the auditory tubes into the pharynx
- Contain **follicles** with **germinal centers**
- Are not fully encapsulated
- Epithelial tissue overlying tonsil masses invaginates, forming **tonsillar crypts**

Crypts trap and destroy bacteria and particulate matter

Aggregates of Lymphoid Follicles
- **Peyer's patches** - Clusters of lymphoid follicles in the wall of the distal portion of the small intestine
- **Peyer's patches in the appendix** - Destroy bacteria, preventing them from breaching the intestinal wall

Generate "memory" lymphocytes

MALT - **M**ucosa-**a**ssociated **l**ymphatic **t**issue protects the digestive and respiratory systems from foreign matter
- Peyer's patches, tonsils, and the appendix (**digestive tract**)

Lymphoid nodules in the walls of the bronchi (respiratory tract)

Immunity

- Resistance to disease
  - **Innate defense system** has two lines of defense
    - **First line of defense** is external body membranes (skin and mucosae)
    - **Second line of defense** is antimicrobial proteins, phagocytes, and other cells
    - Inhibit spread of invaders
  - **Adaptive defense system**
    - Third line of defense attacks particular foreign substances
    - Takes longer to react than the innate system
  - Innate and adaptive defenses are deeply intertwined

Figure 19.4 Complement activation

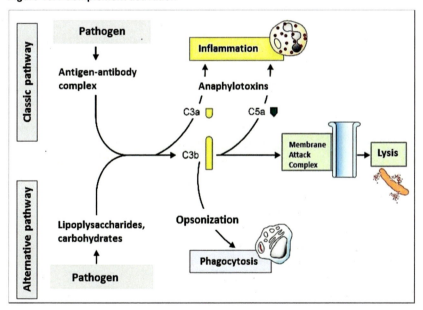

Innate defense system

Surface barriers - Skin, mucous membranes, and their secretions
- **Physical barrier** to most microorganisms
- **Protective chemicals** inhibit or destroy microorganisms
  - Skin acidity; lipids in sebum and dermcidin in sweat; HCl and protein-digesting enzymes of stomach mucosae; lysozyme of saliva and lacrimal fluid, mucus
- **Respiratory system modifications**

- Mucus-coated hairs in the nose
- Cilia of upper respiratory tract sweep dust- and bacteria-laden mucus from lower respiratory passages

Internal Defenses: Cells and Chemicals
- Necessary if microorganisms invade deeper tissues

Phagocytes	• **Macrophages** develop from monocytes to become the chief phagocytic cells
	  • **Free macrophages** wander through tissue spaces, e. g., alveolar macrophages
	  • **Fixed macrophages** are permanent residents of some organs, e. g., Kupffer cells (liver) and microglia (brain)
	• **Neutrophils** become phagocytic on encountering infectious material in tissues
	• **Mechanism of Phagocytosis**
	  • Adherence of phagocyte to pathogen
	  • Pseudopods engulf the particles forming a **phagosome**
	  • Lysosome fuses with the phagosome → **phagolysosome**
	  • Lysosomal enzymes digest pathogen, leaving a residual body.
	  • Exocytosis removes indigestible and residual material

Natural Killer (NK) Cells	• Large granular lymphocytes • Target cells that lack "self" cell-surface receptors • Induce apoptosis in cancer cells and virus-infected cells • Secrete potent chemicals that enhance the inflammatory response

Inflammatory Response	• Triggered whenever body tissues are injured or infected
	• Prevents the spread of damaging agents
	• Disposes of cell debris and pathogens
	• Sets the stage for repair
	• **Cardinal signs of acute inflammation**:
	  • Redness
	  • Heat
	  • Swelling
	  • Pain
	  • (And sometimes Impairment of function)
	• **Inflammatory mediators** released by injured tissue, phagocytes, lymphocytes, basophils, and mast cells
	  • Histamine (from mast cells)
	  • Blood proteins
	  • Kinins, prostaglandins (PGs), leukotrienes, and

	complement
	• Inflammatory chemicals cause
	  • Dilation of arterioles, resulting in **hyperemia**
	  • Increased permeability of local capillaries and **edema** (leakage of exudate)
	  • Exudate contains proteins, clotting factors, and antibodies
	  • Moves foreign material into lymphatic vessels
	  • Delivers clotting proteins to form a scaffold for repair and to isolate the area
	• **Phagocyte Mobilization** - Neutrophils, then phagocytes flood to inflamed sites
	• **Steps for phagocyte mobilization**
	  • **Leukocytosis**: release of neutrophils from bone marrow in response to leukocytosis-inducing factors from injured cells
	  • **Margination**: neutrophils cling to the walls of capillaries in the inflamed area
	  • **Diapedesis** of neutrophils
	  • **Chemotaxis**: inflammatory chemicals promote positive chemotaxis of neutrophils

Antimicrobial Proteins	• Attack microorganisms directly
	• Hinder microorganisms' ability to reproduce
	• **Interferons**
	  • Viral-infected cells are activated to secrete IFNs
	  • IFNs enter neighboring cells
	  • Neighboring cells produce antiviral proteins that block viral reproduction
	  • Produced by a variety of body cells
	  • Interferons also activate macrophages and mobilize NKs
	  • **Functions**: Anti-viral, reduce inflammation, activate macrophages and mobilize NK cells
	  • **Genetically engineered IFNs** for
	    • Antiviral agents against hepatitis and genital warts virus
	    • Multiple sclerosis treatment
	• **Complement** - Major mechanism for destroying foreign substances
	  • ~20 blood proteins that circulate in an inactive form
	  • Amplifies all aspects of the inflammatory response
	  • Kills bacteria and certain other cell types by cell lysis
	  • Enhances both nonspecific and specific defenses
	  • **Complement Activation**
	    • **Classical pathway** - Antibodies bind to invading organisms

	• C1 binds to the antigen-antibody complexes (**complement fixation**)
	• **Alternative pathway** - Triggered when activated C3, B, D, and P interact on the surface of microorganisms
	• Each pathway involves activation of proteins in an orderly sequence
	• Both pathways converge on C3, which cleaves into C3a and C3b
	• **Activated complement**
	  • Enhances inflammation
	  • Promotes phagocytosis
	  • C3b initiates formation of a **membrane attack complex** (MAC) → **cell lysis** by inducing a massive influx of water
	  • **C3b** also causes **opsonization**, and **C3a** causes **inflammation**

Fever	• Systemic response to invading microorganisms
	• Leukocytes and macrophages exposed to foreign substances secrete pyrogens
	• Pyrogens reset the body's thermostat upward
	• Benefits of moderate fever
	  • Causes the liver and spleen to sequester iron and zinc
	  • Increases metabolic rate, which speeds up repair
	• High fevers are dangerous because heat denatures enzymes

Adaptive defense system

- Protects against infectious agents and abnormal body cells
- Amplifies the inflammatory response
- Activates complement
- Is specific, is systemic, has memory
- Two separate overlapping arms
  - **Humoral (antibody-mediated) immunity**
  - **Cellular (cell-mediated) immunity**
- Uses lymphocytes, APCs, and specific molecules to identify and destroy nonself substances
- Depends upon the ability of its cells to
  - Recognize antigens by binding to them
  - Communicate with one another so that the whole system mounts a specific response

Antigens - Substances that can mobilize the adaptive defenses and provoke an immune response
- Most are large, complex molecules not normally found in the body (nonself)
- **Complete Antigens**, e.g., foreign protein, polysaccharides, lipids, and nucleic acids

- Important functional properties
  - **Immunogenicity**: ability to stimulate proliferation of specific lymphocytes and antibodies
  - **Reactivity**: ability to react with products of activated lymphocytes and antibodies released
- **Haptens (Incomplete Antigens)** - Small molecules (peptides, nucleotides, and hormones)
  - Not immunogenic by themselves, but immunogenic when attached to body proteins
  - **Cause the immune system to mount a harmful attack**; e.g., poison ivy, animal dander, detergents, and cosmetics
- **Antigenic Determinants (epitopes)** - Certain parts of an entire antigen that are immunogenic
  - Antibodies and lymphocyte receptors bind to them
  - Most naturally occurring antigens have numerous antigenic determinants that
  - Mobilize several different lymphocyte populations
  - Form different kinds of antibodies against it
  - Large, chemically simple molecules (e.g., plastics) have little or no immunogenicity

Self-Antigens: MHC Proteins
- Protein molecules (self-antigens) on the surface of cells
- Antigenic to others in transfusions or grafts
- Coded for by genes of the **major histocompatibility complex** (MHC) and are unique to an individual
- **Classes of MHC proteins**
  - **Class I MHC proteins**, found on virtually all body cells
  - **Class II MHC proteins**, found on certain cells in the immune response

Cells of the Adaptive Immune System
- Two types of **lymphocytes**
  - **B lymphocytes** (B cells) - humoral immunity
  - **T lymphocytes** (T cells) - cell-mediated immunity
- **Antigen-presenting cells** (APCs)
  - Do not respond to specific antigens
  - Play essential auxiliary roles in immunity

Lymphocytes - Originate in red bone marrow
- **B cells** mature in the red bone marrow
- **T cells** mature in the thymus
- When mature, they have
  - **Immunocompetence**; they are able to recognize and bind to a specific antigen
  - **Self-tolerance** – unresponsive to self-antigens
- Naive (unexposed) B and T cells are exported to lymph nodes, spleen, and other lymphoid organs
- **T Cells** mature in the thymus under negative and positive selection pressures
  - **Positive selection**: Selects T cells capable of binding to self-MHC proteins (MHC restriction)
  - **Negative selection**: Prompts apoptosis of T cells that bind to self-antigens displayed by self-MHC

- Ensures self-tolerance
- **B cells** mature in red bone marrow
  - Self-reactive B cells
    - Are eliminated by apoptosis (clonal deletion) or
    - Undergo receptor editing – rearrangement of their receptors
    - Are inactivated (anergy) if they escape from the bone marrow
- **Antigen-Presenting Cells** (APCs) - Present fragments of antigens to be recognized by T cells
  - Major types
    - **Dendritic cells** in connective tissues and epidermis
    - **Macrophages** in connective tissues and lymphoid organs
    - **B cells**
  - Macrophages and Dendritic Cells present antigens and activate T cells
  - Macrophages mostly remain fixed in the lymphoid organs
  - Activated T cells release chemicals that prod macrophages to become insatiable phagocytes and to secrete bactericidal chemicals
  - Dendritic cells internalize pathogens and enter lymphatics to present the antigens to T cells in lymphoid organs

Humoral Immunity Response

Antigen challenge - First encounter between an antigen and a naive immunocompetent lymphocyte
- Usually occurs in the spleen or a lymph node
- If the lymphocyte is a **B cell**
  - The antigen provokes a **humoral immune response**
  - **Antibodies** are produced

Clonal Selection - B cell is activated when antigens bind to its surface receptors and cross-link them
- **Stimulated B cell** grows to **form a clone** of identical cells bearing the same antigen-specific receptors (T helper cells usually required to achieve full activation)
- Most clone cells become **plasma cells** that **secrete specific antibodies** at the rate of 2000 molecules per second for four to five days
- Clone cells that do not become plasma cells become **memory cells**
  - Provide immunological memory
  - Mount an immediate response to future exposures of the same antigen

Immunological Memory
- **Primary immune response** - Occurs on the **first exposure** to a specific antigen
  - **Lag period**: three to six days
  - Peak levels of plasma antibody are reached in 10 days
  - Antibody levels then decline
- **Secondary immune response** - Occurs on **re-exposure to the same antigen**
  - Sensitized memory cells respond within hours
  - Antibody levels peak in two to three days at much higher levels
  - Antibodies bind with greater affinity
  - Antibody level can remain high for weeks to months

- **Active Humoral Immunity** - Occurs when B cells encounter antigens and produce specific antibodies against them
  - **Naturally acquired** - response to a bacterial or viral infection
  - **Artificially acquired** - response to a vaccine of dead or attenuated pathogens
  - **Vaccines** spare us the symptoms of the primary response
    - Provide antigenic determinants that are immunogenic and reactive
    - Target only one type of helper T cell, so fail to fully establish cellular immunological memory
- **Passive Humoral Immunity**
  - B cells are not challenged by antigens
  - Immunological memory does not occur
  - **Naturally acquired** - antibodies delivered to a fetus via the placenta or to infant through milk
  - **Artificially acquired** - injection of serum, such as gamma globulin
    - Protection is immediate but ends when antibodies naturally degrade in the body

Figure 19.5 Primary and secondary immune response

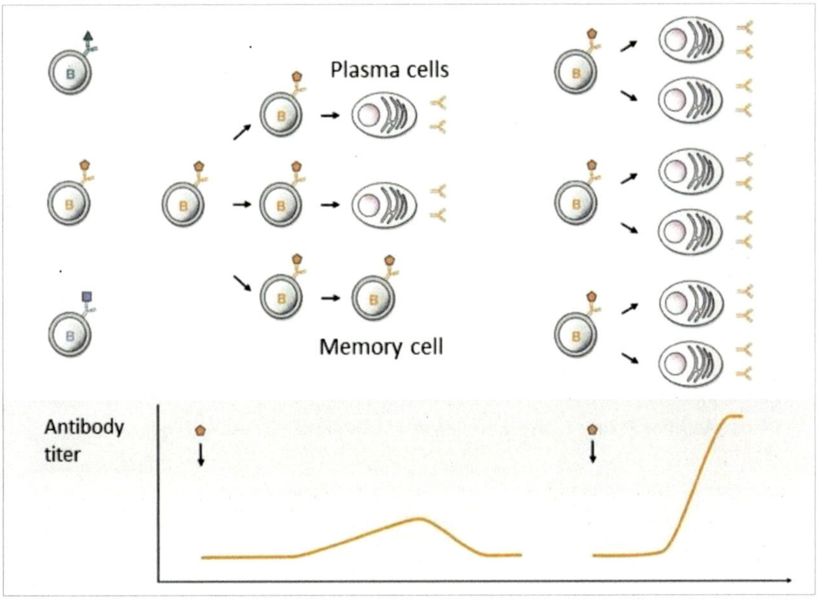

Antibodies
- **Immunoglobulins** - **gamma globulin** portion of blood proteins secreted by plasma cells
- **Basic Antibody Structure**
  - T-or Y-shaped monomer of four looping linked polypeptide chains
  - Two identical **heavy (H) chains** and two identical **light (L) chains**
  - **Variable (V) regions** of each arm combine to form two identical antigen-binding sites
  - **Constant (C) region** of stem determines

- The antibody class (IgM, IgA, IgD, IgG, or IgE)
- The cells and chemicals that the antibody can bind to
- How the antibody class functions in antigen elimination
- **IgM** - A pentamer; first antibody released; potent agglutinating agent; readily fixes and activates complement
- **IgA** (secretory IgA) - Monomer or dimer; in mucus and other secretions; helps prevent entry of pathogens
- **IgD** - Monomer attached to the surface of B cells; functions as a B cell receptor
- **IgG** - Monomer; 75–85% of antibodies in plasma; from secondary and late primary responses; crosses the placental barrier
- **IgE** - Monomer active in some allergies and parasitic infections; causes mast cells and basophils to release histamine

Antibody Diversity
- Billions of antibodies result from somatic recombination of gene segments
- **Hypervariable regions** of some genes increase antibody variation through somatic mutations
- Each plasma cell can switch the type of H chain produced, making an antibody of a different class

- **Antibodies inactivate and tag antigens**
- Form antigen-antibody (immune) complexes
- Defensive mechanisms used by antibodies:
  - **Neutralization** - Antibodies block specific sites on viruses or bacterial exotoxins
    - Prevent these antigens from binding to receptors on tissue cells
    - Antigen-antibody complexes undergo phagocytosis
  - **Agglutination** - Antibodies bind the same determinant on more than one cell-bound antigen
    - Cross-linked antigen-antibody complexes agglutinate; e.g., clumping of mismatched blood cells
  - **Precipitation** - Soluble molecules are cross-linked
    - Complexes precipitate and are subject to phagocytosis
  - **Complement Fixation and Activation** - Main antibody defense against cellular antigens
    - Several antibodies bind close together on a cellular antigen
    - Their complement-binding sites trigger complement fixation into the cell's surface
    - Complement triggers cell lysis
    - Amplifies the inflammatory response
    - Opsonization
    - Enlists more and more defensive elements

Monoclonal Antibodies
- Commercially prepared pure antibody
  - Produced by **hybridomas - cell hybrids**: fusion of a tumor cell and a B cell
  - Proliferate indefinitely and have the ability to produce a single type of antibody
- Used in research, clinical testing, and cancer treatment

Cell-Mediated Immune Response

- T cells provide defense against intracellular antigens
- Two types of surface receptors of T cells
  - T cell antigen receptors
  - Cell differentiation glycoproteins CD4 or CD8
- Play a role in T cell interactions with other cells
- Major types of T cells
  - **CD4 cells** become **helper T cells** (TH) when activated
  - **CD8 cells** become **cytotoxic T cells** (TC) that destroy cells harboring foreign antigens
- Other types of T cells
  - **Regulatory T cells** (TREG)
  - **Memory T cells**

Antigen Recognition - Immunocompetent T cells are activated when their surface receptors bind to a recognized antigen (nonself)
- T cells must simultaneously recognize **Nonself** (antigen) and **Self** (MHC protein)
- **MHC Proteins**
  - **Class I MHC proteins** - displayed by all cells except RBCs
  - **Class II MHC proteins** – displayed by APCs (dendritic cells, macrophages and B cells)
  - Both types are synthesized at the ER and bind to peptide fragments
  - **Class I MHC Proteins** - Bind with fragment of a protein synthesized in the cell **(endogenous antigen)**
    - Endogenous antigen is a self-antigen in a normal cell; a nonself antigen in an infected or abnormal cell
    - Informs **cytotoxic T cells** of the presence of microorganisms hiding in cells
  - **Class II MHC Proteins** - Bind with fragments of exogenous antigens that have been engulfed and broken down in a phagolysosome
    - Recognized by **helper T cells**

T Cell Activation

- APCs migrate to lymph nodes and other lymphoid tissues to present their antigens to T cells
- T cell activation is a two-step process
  - **Antigen Binding** - CD4 and CD8 cells bind to different classes of MHC proteins **(MHC restriction)**
    - **CD4 cells** bind to antigen linked to **class II MHC** proteins of APCs
    - **CD8 cells** are activated by antigen fragments linked to class **I MHC** of APCs
    - **Dendritic cells** are able to obtain other cells' **endogenous antigens**
  - **Co-Stimulation** - Requires T cell binding to other surface receptors on an APC
    - Cytokines (interleukin 1 and 2 from APCs or T cells) trigger proliferation and differentiation of activated T cell
  - **Without co-stimulation,** anergy occurs; cells become tolerant to that antigen
- **T cells that are activated e**nlarge, proliferate, and form clones
  - Differentiate and perform functions according to their T cell class
  - **Primary T cell response** peaks within a week

- **T cell apoptosis** occurs between days 7 and 30
  - Effector activity wanes as the amount of antigen declines
  - Benefit of apoptosis: activated T cells are a hazard
- **Memory T cells** remain and mediate secondary responses

Cytokines - Mediate cell development, differentiation, and responses in the immune system
- Include **interleukins and interferons**
- Other cytokines amplify and regulate innate and adaptive responses
- Some **chemotactic cytokines** or **chemokines** are used in the treatment of viral infections, such as HIV

Helper T (T_H) Cells - Play a central role in the adaptive immune response
- Help activate T and B cells and induce T and B cell proliferation
- Activate macrophages and recruit other immune cells
- Stimulate B cells to divide more rapidly and begin antibody formation
- Most antigens require T_H co-stimulation to activate B cells
- Cause dendritic cells to express co-stimulatory molecules required for CD8 cell activation
- **Without T_H, there is no immune response**

Cytotoxic T (T_C) Cells - Directly attack and kill other cells
- Activated T_C cells circulate in blood and lymph and lymphoid organs in search of body cells displaying antigen they recognize
  - **Targets:** Virus-infected cells, cells with intracellular bacteria or parasites, cancer cells, foreign cells (transfusions or transplants)
- **Cytotoxic T Cells bind to a self-nonself complex**
  - Can destroy all **infected or abnormal cells**
    - Tc cell releases perforins and granzymes by exocytosis
    - Perforins create pores through which granzymes enter the target cell
    - Granzymes stimulate apoptosis
    - In some cases, TC cell stimulates apoptosis

Natural Killer Cells - Recognize other signs of abnormality
- Lack of class I MHC
- Antibody coating a target cell
- Different surface marker on stressed cells
- Use the same key mechanisms as Tc cells for killing their target cells

Regulatory T (T_{Reg}) Cells - Dampen the immune response by direct contact or by inhibitory cytokines
- Important in preventing autoimmune reactions

Comparison of Humoral and Cell-Mediated Response
- **Antibodies** of the **humoral response** - The simplest ammunition of the immune response; **Targets:** Bacteria and molecules in extracellular environments (body secretions, tissue fluid, blood, and lymph)
- **T cells** of the **cell-mediated response** - Recognize and respond only to processed fragments of antigen displayed on the surface of body cells; **Targets:** Body cells infected by viruses or bacteria, abnormal or cancerous cells, cells of infused or transplanted foreign tissue

A&P Essentials 4th ed.

Figure 19.6 Innate and adaptive defense system

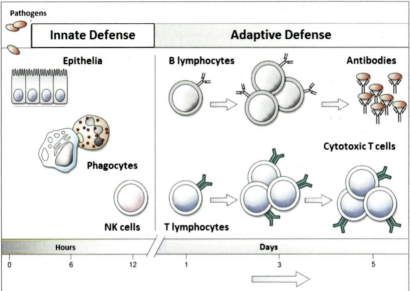

Organ Transplants

- **Autografts**: from one body site to another in the same person
- **Isografts**: between identical twins
- **Allografts**: between individuals who are not identical twins
- **Xenografts**: from another animal species

Hypersensitivities - Immune responses to a perceived (otherwise harmless) threat
- Causes tissue damage
- Different types are distinguished by
  - Their time course
  - Whether antibodies or T cells are involved
    - **Antibodies** cause **immediate and subacute hypersensitivities**
    - **T cells** cause **delayed hypersensitivity**
- **Immediate Hypersensitivity**
  - **Acute (type I) hypersensitivities** (allergies) begin in seconds after contact with allergen; reaction may be local or systemic; IgE binds to mast cells and basophils, resulting in a flood of histamine release and inducing the inflammatory response
  - **Anaphylactic Shock** - Systemic response to allergen that directly enters the blood
    - Systemic histamine releases may cause constriction of bronchioles, sudden vasodilation and fluid loss from the bloodstream, hypotensive shock and death
    - **Treatment:** epinephrine
- **Subacute Hypersensitivities** - Caused by IgM and IgG transferred via blood plasma or serum; slow onset (1–3 hours) and long duration (10–15 hours)
  - **Cytotoxic (type II) reactions** - Antibodies bind to antigens on specific body cells,

stimulating phagocytosis and complement-mediated lysis of the cellular antigens
- **Immune complex (type III) hypersensitivity** - Antigens are widely distributed through the body or blood
  - Insoluble antigen-antibody complexes form
  - Complexes cannot be cleared from a particular area of the body
  - Intense inflammation, local cell lysis, and death may result
- **Delayed Hypersensitivities (Type IV)** - Slow onset (one to three days)
  - Mechanism depends on helper T cells
  - Cytokine-activated macrophages and cytotoxic T cells cause damage

Chapter 20 Respiratory System

Respiration

- Involves both the respiratory and the circulatory systems
- Four processes that supply the body with O_2 and dispose of CO_2
  - **Pulmonary ventilation** (breathing): movement of air into and out of the lungs
  - **External respiration**: O_2 and CO_2 exchange between the lungs and the blood
  - **Transport**: O_2 and CO_2 in the blood
  - **Internal respiration**: O_2 and CO_2 exchange between systemic blood vessels and tissues

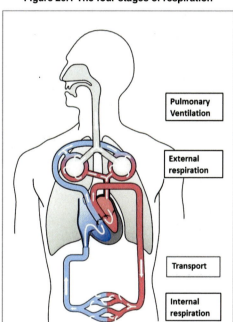

Figure 20.1 The four stages of respiration

Functional Anatomy

Respiratory zone: Site of gas exchange
- **Microscopic structures**: respiratory bronchioles, alveolar ducts, and alveoli

Conducting zone: Conduits to gas exchange sites
- Includes all other respiratory structures

Respiratory muscles: Diaphragm and other muscles that promote ventilation

Nose, nasal cavity and paranasal sinuses
- Provide airway for respiration
- Filter, heat, and moisten air
- Serve as a resonating chamber for speech
- Reclaim heat and moisture during exhalation
- Houses olfactory receptors

- **External nose**: root, bridge, dorsum nasi, and apex (tip)
  - **Philtrum**: a shallow vertical groove inferior to the apex
  - **Nostrils** (nares): bounded laterally by the alae
- **Nasal cavity**: in and posterior to the external nose; divided by a midline **nasal septum**
  - **Posterior nasal apertures** (choanae) open into the nasal pharynx
  - **Roof**: ethmoid and sphenoid bones
  - **Floor**: hard and soft palates
  - **Vestibule**: nasal cavity superior to the nostrils
  - **Vibrissae** filter coarse particles from inspired air
  - **Olfactory mucosa** - Lines the superior nasal cavity; contains smell receptors
  - **Respiratory mucosa** - Mucous and serous secretions contain lysozyme and defensins
    - Cilia move contaminated mucus posteriorly to throat
    - Inspired air is warmed by plexuses of capillaries and veins
    - Sensory nerve endings triggers sneezing
  - **Superior, middle, and inferior nasal conchae** - Protrude from the lateral walls
    - Increase mucosal area
    - Enhance air turbulence
- **Paranasal Sinuses** - In frontal, sphenoid, ethmoid, and maxillary bones
  - Lighten the skull and help to warm and moisten the air

Figure 20.2 Upper airways

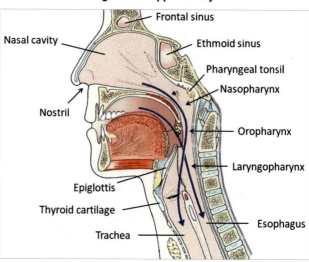

- **Pharynx** - Muscular tube that connects to the
  - Nasal cavity and mouth superiorly
  - Larynx and esophagus inferiorly
  - From the base of the skull to the level of the sixth cervical vertebra
- **Nasopharynx** - Air passageway posterior to the nasal cavity

- **Soft palate and uvula** close nasopharynx during swallowing
- **Pharyngeal tonsil** (adenoids) on posterior wall
- **Pharyngotympanic** (auditory) **tubes** open into the lateral walls
- **Oropharynx** - Passageway for food and air from the level of the soft palate to the epiglottis
  - **Isthmus of the fauces**: opening to the oral cavity
  - **Palatine tonsils** in the lateral walls of fauces
  - **Lingual tonsil** on the posterior surface of the tongue
- **Laryngopharynx** - Passageway for food and air
  - Posterior to the upright epiglottis
  - Extends to the larynx, where it is also continuous with the esophagus

Larynx
- Attaches to the hyoid bone and opens into the laryngopharynx; continuous with the trachea
- Provides a patent airway; routes air and food into proper channels; voice production
- **Cartilages of the larynx** - Hyaline cartilage except for the epiglottis
  - **Thyroid cartilage** with **laryngeal prominence** (Adam's apple)
  - Ring-shaped **cricoid cartilage**
  - Paired **arytenoid, cuneiform**, and **corniculate cartilages**
  - **Epiglottis**: elastic cartilage; covers the laryngeal inlet during swallowing
- **Vocal ligaments** - Attach the arytenoid cartilages to the thyroid cartilage
  - Contain elastic fibers
  - Form core of **vocal folds** (true vocal cords)
  - Opening between them is the **glottis**
  - Folds vibrate to produce sound as air rushes up from the lungs
- **Vestibular folds** (false vocal cords) - Superior to the vocal folds
  - No part in sound production
  - Help to close the glottis during swallowing

Trachea (Windpipe): From the larynx into the mediastinum
- **Trachealis muscle** - Connects posterior parts of cartilage rings
  - Contracts during coughing to expel mucus
- **Carina** - Last tracheal cartilage
  - Point where trachea branches into two bronchi

Bronchi undergo 23 orders of branching
- Branching pattern called the **bronchial (respiratory) tree**
  - **Trachea** → right and left **main (primary) bronchi** → **lobar (secondary) bronchi** (three right, two left) → **segmental (tertiary) bronchi** (divide repeatedly)
  - **Bronchioles** are less than 1 mm in diameter
  - **Terminal bronchioles** are the smallest, less than 0.5 mm diameter

Conducting Zone Structures
- From bronchi through bronchioles, structural changes occur
  - Cartilage rings give way to plates; cartilage is absent from bronchioles
  - Epithelium changes from pseudostratified columnar to cuboidal; cilia and goblet cells become sparse

- Relative amount of smooth muscle increases

Respiratory Zone
- Respiratory bronchioles, alveolar ducts, alveolar sacs (clusters of alveoli)
- ~300 million alveoli account for most of the lungs' volume and are the main site for gas exchange
- **Alveoli**
  - Surrounded by fine elastic fibers
  - Contain open pores that connect adjacent alveoli
  - Allow air pressure throughout the lung to be equalized
  - House alveolar macrophages that keep alveolar surfaces sterile
  - **Respiratory Membrane**
    - ~0.5-μm-thick air-blood barrier
    - Alveolar and capillary walls and their fused basement membranes
  - **Alveolar walls** - Single layer of squamous epithelium (**type I cells**)
  - Scattered **type II** cuboidal **cells** secrete surfactant and antimicrobial proteins

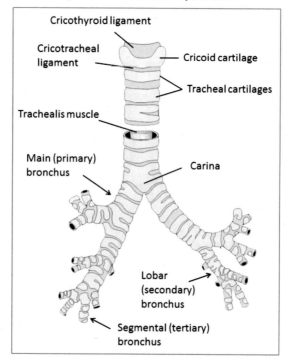

Figure 20.3 Trachea and major bronchi

Lungs

- **Root**: site of vascular and bronchial attachments
- **Costal surface**: anterior, lateral, and posterior surfaces
- **Apex**: superior tip
- **Base**: inferior surface that rests on the diaphragm
- **Hilum**: on mediastinal surface; site for attachment of blood vessels, bronchi, lymphatic

vessels, and nerves
- **Cardiac notch of left lung**: concavity that accommodates the heart
- **Left lung** is smaller, separated into two lobes by an oblique fissure
- **Right lung** has three lobes separated by oblique and horizontal fissures
- **Bronchopulmonary segments** (10 right, 8–9 left)
- **Lobules** are the smallest subdivisions; served by bronchioles and their branches

Blood Supply
- **Pulmonary circulation** (low pressure, high volume)
  - Pulmonary arteries deliver systemic venous blood; feed into the pulmonary capillary networks; pulmonary veins carry oxygenated blood from respiratory zones to the heart
- **Systemic circulation** (high pressure, low volume)
  - Bronchial arteries provide oxygenated blood to lung tissue; arise from aorta and enter the lungs at the hilum; supply all lung tissue except the alveoli
  - Bronchial veins anastomose with pulmonary veins; pulmonary veins carry most venous blood back to the heart

Pleurae - Thin, double-layered serosa
- **Parietal pleura** on thoracic wall and superior face of diaphragm
- **Visceral pleura** on external lung surface
- Pleural fluid fills the slit-like **pleural cavity**
  - Provides lubrication and surface tension

Figure 20.4 Lungs and pleura

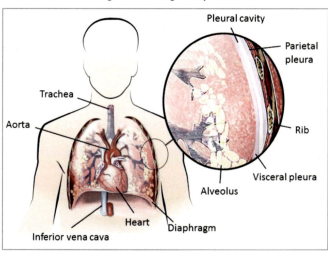

Mechanics of Breathing

Pressure Relationships in the Thoracic Cavity
- **Atmospheric pressure** (P_{atm}): Pressure exerted by the air surrounding the body; 760 mm Hg at sea level
- **Respiratory pressures** are described relative to P_{atm}
  - Negative respiratory pressure is less than P_{atm}, positive respiratory pressure greater

- Zero respiratory pressure = P_{atm}
- **Intrapulmonary (intra-alveolar) pressure** (P_{pul}): Pressure in the alveoli; fluctuates with breathing; always eventually equalizes with P_{atm}
- **Intrapleural pressure** (P_{ip}): Pressure in the pleural cavity; fluctuates with breathing
  - Always a negative pressure (<P_{atm} and <P_{pul})
  - Negative P_{ip} is caused by opposing forces
    - **Elastic recoil** of lungs decreases lung size
    - **Surface tension** of alveolar fluid reduces alveolar size
    - Elasticity of the chest wall pulls the thorax outward
- **Transpulmonary pressure** = ($P_{pul} - P_{ip}$): Keeps the airways open
  - The greater the transpulmonary pressure, the larger the lungs
  - If $P_{ip} = P_{pul}$ the lungs collapse
  - **Atelectasis** (lung collapse) is due to
  - Plugged bronchioles → collapse of alveoli
  - Wound that admits air into pleural cavity (**pneumothorax**)

Pulmonary ventilation consists of two phases
- **Inspiration**: gases flow into the lungs
- **Expiration**: gases exit the lungs
- Mechanical processes that depend on volume changes in the thoracic cavity
  - Volume changes → pressure changes
  - Pressure changes → gases flow to equalize pressure
- **Boyle's Law** - The relationship between the pressure and volume of a gas
  - Pressure (*P*) varies inversely with volume (*V*): $P_1V_1 = P_2V_2$

Inspiration – Always an active process
- Inspiratory muscles contract → thoracic volume increases → lungs are stretched and intrapulmonary volume increases → intrapulmonary pressure drops (to −1 mm Hg) → air flows into the lungs, down its pressure gradient, until $P_{pul} = P_{atm}$

Expiration - Quiet expiration is normally a passive process
- Inspiratory muscles relax → thoracic cavity volume decreases → elastic lungs recoil and intrapulmonary volume decreases → P_{pul} rises (to +1 mm Hg) → air flows out of the lungs down its pressure gradient until Ppul = 0
- **Forced expiration is an active process**: it uses abdominal and internal intercostal muscles

Physical Factors Influencing Pulmonary Ventilation
- Inspiratory muscles consume energy to overcome three factors that hinder air passage and pulmonary ventilation
- **Airway** Resistance - Friction is the major nonelastic source of resistance to gas flow
  - **Gas flow changes inversely with resistance**
  - **Resistance is usually insignificant**
  - As airway resistance rises, breathing movements become more strenuous
    - Severely constricting or obstruction of bronchioles
    - Can prevent life-sustaining ventilation
    - Can occur during acute asthma attacks and stop ventilation
    - Epinephrine dilates bronchioles and reduces air resistance
- **Alveolar Surface Tension**

- **Surface tension** attracts liquid molecules to one another at a gas-liquid interface
  - Resists any force that tends to increase the surface area of the liquid
- **Surfactant:** Detergent-like lipid and protein complex produced by type II alveolar cells
  - Reduces surface tension of alveolar fluid and discourages alveolar collapse
  - Insufficient quantity in premature infants causes infant respiratory distress syndrome
- **Lung Compliance** - A measure of the change in lung volume that occurs with a given change in transpulmonary pressure
  - Normally high due to
    - Distensibility of the lung tissue
    - Alveolar surface tension
  - Diminished by
    - Nonelastic scar tissue (fibrosis)
    - Reduced production of surfactant
    - Decreased flexibility of the thoracic cage
  - **Homeostatic imbalances** that reduce compliance
    - Deformities of thorax
    - Ossification of the costal cartilage
    - Paralysis of intercostal muscles

Respiratory Volumes and Capacities

Tidal volume (TV)	Amount of air inhaled or exhaled with each breath under resting conditions
Inspiratory reserve volume (IRV)	Amount of air that can be forcefully inhaled after a normal tidal volume inhalation
Expiratory reserve volume (ERV)	Amount of air that can be forcefully exhaled after a normal tidal volume exhalation
Residual volume (RV)	Amount of air remaining in the lungs after forced exhalation
Inspiratory capacity (IC)	Maximum amount of air that can be inspired after a normal expiration: IC = TV + IRV
Functional residual capacity (FRC)	Volume of air remaining in the lungs after a normal tidal volume expiration: FRC = ERV + RV
Vital capacity (VC)	Maximum amount of air that can be expired after a maximum inspiratory effort: VC = TV + IRV + ERV
Total lung capacity (TLC)	Maximum amount of air contained in lungs after a maximum inspiratory effort: TLC = TV + IRV + ERV + RV

Pulmonary Function Tests can distinguish between
- **Obstructive pulmonary disease** - increased airway resistance (e.g., bronchitis)
- **Restrictive pulmonary disorder** - reduction in total lung capacity due to structural or functional lung changes (e.g., fibrosis or TB)
- **Minute ventilation**: total amount of gas flow into or out of the respiratory tract in one minute
- **Forced vital capacity** (FVC): gas forcibly expelled after taking a deep breath

- **Forced expiratory volume** (FEV): the amount of gas expelled during specific time intervals of the FVC

Dead Space - Some inspired air never contributes to gas exchange
- **Anatomical dead space**: volume of the conducting zone conduits (~150 ml)
- **Alveolar dead space**: alveoli that cease to act in gas exchange due to collapse or obstruction
- **Total dead space**: sum of above nonuseful volumes

Alveolar Ventilation

- **Alveolar ventilation rate** (AVR): flow of gases into and out of the alveoli during a particular time
  - Dead space is normally constant
  - Rapid, shallow breathing decreases AVR

Figure 20.5 Lung Volumes and Capacities

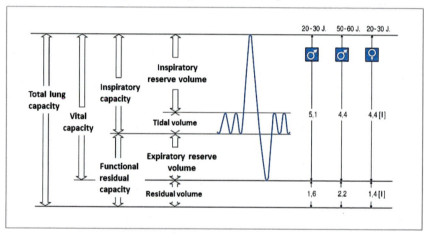

External & Internal Respiration

- **Dalton's Law of Partial Pressures** - Total pressure exerted by a mixture of gases is the sum of the pressures exerted by each gas
  - The **partial pressure** of each gas is directly proportional to its percentage in the mixture
- **Henry's Law** - When a mixture of gases is in contact with a liquid, each gas will dissolve in the liquid in proportion to its partial pressure
  - At equilibrium, the partial pressures in the two phases will be equal
- The amount of gas that will dissolve in a liquid also depends upon its solubility
  - CO_2 is 20 times more soluble in water than O_2

Composition of Alveolar Gas
- Alveoli contain more CO_2 and water vapor than atmospheric air, due to
  - Gas exchanges in the lungs
  - Humidification of air

- Mixing of alveolar gas that occurs with each breath

External Respiration - Exchange of O_2 and CO_2 across the respiratory membrane
- **Partial pressure gradient for O_2** in the lungs is steep
  - **Venous blood Po_2** = 40 mm Hg
  - **Alveolar Po_2** = 104 mm Hg
  - O_2 partial pressures reach equilibrium of 104 mm Hg in ~0.25 seconds, about 1/3 the time a red blood cell is in a pulmonary capillary
- **Partial pressure gradient for CO_2** in the lungs is less steep:
  - **Venous blood Pco_2** = 45 mm Hg
  - **Alveolar Pco_2** = 40 mm Hg
  - CO_2 is 20 times more soluble than oxygen → CO_2 diffuses in equal amounts with oxygen
- **Ventilation-Perfusion Coupling**: Ventilation and perfusion must be matched (coupled) for efficient gas exchange
  - **Ventilation**: amount of gas reaching the alveoli
  - **Perfusion**: blood flow reaching the alveoli
  - **Changes in Po_2** in the alveoli cause changes in the diameters of the arterioles
    - Alveolar O_2 ↑ → arterioles dilate; alveolar O_2 ↓ → arterioles constrict
  - **Changes in Pco_2** in the alveoli cause changes in the diameters of the bronchioles
    - Alveolar CO_2 ↑ → bronchioles dilate; alveolar CO_2 ↓ → bronchioles constrict
- **Respiratory membrane**
  - 0.5 to 1 μm thick - Thickens if lungs become waterlogged and edematous, and gas exchange becomes inadequate
  - Large **total surface area** (40 times that of one's skin) - Reduction in surface area with emphysema, when walls of adjacent alveoli break down

Internal Respiration - Capillary gas exchange in body tissues
- Partial pressures and diffusion gradients are reversed compared to external respiration
- Po_2 in tissue is always lower than in systemic arterial blood; Po_2 of venous blood is 40 mm Hg and Pco_2 is 45 mm Hg
- O_2 moves from blood into tissue; CO_2 moves from tissue into blood

Gas Transport in the Blood

O_2 Transport - Molecular O_2 is carried in the blood
- 1.5% dissolved in plasma
- 98.5% loosely bound to each Fe of hemoglobin (Hb) in RBCs
- **Oxyhemoglobin** (HbO_2): hemoglobin-O_2 combination
- **Deoxyhemoglobin** or **reduced hemoglobin** (HHb): hemoglobin that has released O_2
- Loading and unloading of O_2 is facilitated by change in shape of Hb
  - O_2 binds, Hb affinity for O_2 increases - O_2 is released, Hb affinity for O_2 decreases
  - **Fully (100%) saturated** if all four heme groups carry O_2
  - **Partially saturated** when one to three heme groups carry O_2
  - Rate of loading and unloading of O_2 is regulated by Po_2, temperature, blood pH,

Pco_2

- **Oxygen-hemoglobin dissociation curve** - S-shaped curve
  - **In arterial blood:** Po_2 = 100 mm Hg; contains 20 ml oxygen per 100 ml blood (20 vol %); Hb is 98% saturated; further increases in Po_2 (e.g., breathing deeply) produce minimal increases in O_2 binding
  - **In venous blood:** Po_2 = 40 mm Hg; contains 15 vol % oxygen; Hb is 75% saturated
  - Hemoglobin is almost completely saturated at a Po_2 of 70 mm Hg → O_2 loading and delivery to tissues is adequate when Po_2 is below normal levels
  - Only 20–25% of bound O_2 is unloaded during one systemic circulation
  - If O_2 levels in tissues drop:
    - More oxygen dissociates from hemoglobin and is used by cells
    - Respiratory rate or cardiac output need not increase
- **Other Factors Influencing Hemoglobin Saturation**
  - Increases in temperature, H^+ and Pco_2 modify the structure of hemoglobin and decrease its affinity for O_2; occur in systemic capillaries; enhance O_2 unloading → shift the O_2-hemoglobin dissociation curve to the right
- **Factors that Increase Release of O_2 by Hemoglobin**
  - As cells metabolize glucose Pco_2 and H^+ increase in concentration in capillary blood
  - Declining pH weakens the hemoglobin-O_2 bond (**Bohr effect**)
  - Increasing temperature directly and indirectly decreases Hb affinity for O_2
  - **Hypoxia:** Inadequate O_2 delivery to tissues due to for example too few RBCs, abnormal or too little Hb, blocked circulation, metabolic poisons, pulmonary disease

Figure 20.6 Carbon dioxide loading in tissues

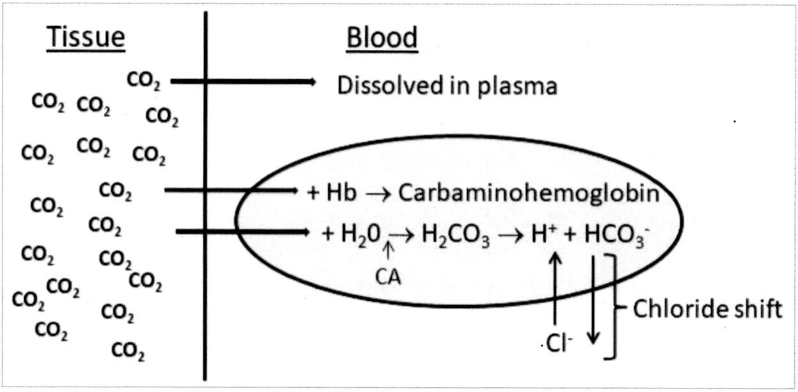

Tissue	Blood
CO_2 CO_2 CO_2 CO_2 CO_2 CO_2 CO_2 CO_2 CO_2 CO_2 CO_2 CO_2 CO_2 CO_2 CO_2 CO_2 CO_2 CO_2	Dissolved in plasma + Hb → Carbaminohemoglobin + H_2O →(CA) H_2CO_3 → H^+ + HCO_3^- ↑ Cl^- ↓ Chloride shift

- **CO_2 Transport**
  - 7 to 10% **dissolved in plasma**
  - 20% **bound to hemoglobin** (carbaminohemoglobin)
  - 70% transported as bicarbonate ions (HCO_3^-) in plasma
- CO_2 combines with water to form carbonic acid (H_2CO_3), which quickly dissociates:
- Most of this occurs in RBCs, where **carbonic anhydrase** reversibly and rapidly catalyzes the reaction
  - In **systemic capillaries** HCO_3^- quickly diffuses from RBCs into the plasma
  - The **chloride shift** occurs: outrush of HCO_3^- from the RBCs is balanced as Cl^-

- moves in from the plasma
- In **pulmonary capillaries** HCO_3^- moves into the RBCs and binds with H^+ to form H_2CO_3
- H_2CO_3 is split by **carbonic anhydrase** into CO_2 and water
- CO_2 diffuses into the alveoli
- **Haldane Effect** - The amount of CO_2 transported is affected by the P_{O_2}
- The lower the P_{O_2} and hemoglobin saturation with O_2, the more CO_2 can be carried in the blood
- At the tissues, as more carbon dioxide enters the blood more oxygen dissociates from hemoglobin (**Bohr effect**)
- As HbO_2 releases O_2, it more readily forms bonds with CO_2 to form carbaminohemoglobin

Control of Respiration

- **Inspiratory neurons** excite the inspiratory muscles via the phrenic and intercostal nerves
- **Expiratory neurons** inhibit the inspiratory neurons
- **Depth of breathing** is determined by how actively the respiratory center stimulates the respiratory muscles
- **Rate** is determined by how long the inspiratory center is active
- Both are modified in response to changing body demands

Influence of P_{CO_2}: Rising CO_2 levels are the most powerful respiratory stimulant
- If P_{CO_2} levels rise (**hypercapnia**), CO_2 accumulates in the brain → CO_2 is hydrated; resulting carbonic acid dissociates, releasing H^+ → H^+ stimulates the central chemoreceptors of the brain stem that synapse with the respiratory regulatory centers, increasing the depth and rate of breathing
- **Hyperventilation**: increased depth and rate of breathing that exceeds the body's need to remove CO_2
  - Causes CO_2 levels to decline (**hypocapnia**)
  - May cause cerebral vasoconstriction and cerebral ischemia

Influence of P_{O_2}. Peripheral chemoreceptors in the aortic and carotid bodies are O_2 sensors
- When excited, they cause the respiratory centers to increase ventilation
- When **arterial P_{O_2} falls below 60 mm Hg**, it becomes the **major stimulus for respiration** (via the peripheral chemoreceptors)

Influence of arterial pH - Can modify respiratory rate and rhythm even if CO_2 and O_2 levels are normal
- Decreased pH may reflect CO_2 retention, accumulation of lactic acid, excess ketone bodies in patients with diabetes mellitus
- Respiratory system attempts to raise the pH by increasing respiratory rate and depth
- Changes in arterial pH resulting from CO_2 retention or metabolic factors act indirectly through the peripheral chemoreceptors

Influence of Higher Brain Centers
- **Hypothalamic controls** modify rate and depth of respiration, e.g., breath holding that occurs in anger or gasping with pain
- **Cortical controls** are direct signals from the cerebral motor cortex that bypass medul-

lary controls, e.g., voluntary breath holding

Pulmonary Irritant Reflexes - Receptors in the bronchioles respond to irritants
- Promote reflexive constriction of air passages
- Receptors in the larger airways mediate the cough and sneeze reflexes

Inflation Reflex - Hering-Breuer Reflex
- Stretch receptors in the pleurae and airways are stimulated by lung inflation
- Inhibitory signals to the respiratory centers end inhalation and allow expiration to occur
- Acts more as a protective response than a normal regulatory mechanism

Respiratory Adjustments
- **Exercise:** Adjustments are geared to both the intensity and duration of exercise
  - **Hyperpnea** - Increase in ventilation (10 to 20 fold) in response to metabolic needs
- **High Altitude** - Quick travel to altitudes above 8000 feet may produce symptoms of **acute mountain sickness** (AMS) such as headaches, shortness of breath, nausea, and dizziness; in severe cases, lethal cerebral and pulmonary edema
- **Acclimatization:** respiratory and hematopoietic adjustments to altitude
  - Chemoreceptors become more responsive to P_{CO_2} when P_{O_2} declines
  - Minute ventilation increases and stabilizes in a few days to 2–3 l/min higher
  - Decline in blood O_2 → kidneys ↑ EPO release → RBC numbers ↑ slowly to provide long-term compensation

Chapter 21 Digestive System

Overview

- **Alimentary canal (gastrointestinal or GI tract)** - Digests and absorbs food
  - Mouth, pharynx, esophagus, stomach, small intestine, and large intestine
- **Accessory digestive organs**
  - Teeth, tongue, gallbladder, digestive glands, salivary glands, liver, pancreas

Peritoneum and Peritoneal Cavity
- **Peritoneum**: serous membrane of the abdominal cavity
  - **Visceral peritoneum** on external surface of most digestive organs
  - **Parietal peritoneum** lines the body wall
- **Peritoneal cavity** - Between the two peritoneums; fluid lubricates mobile organs
- **Mesentery** - Double layer of peritoneum; routes for blood vessels, lymphatics, and nerves; holds organs in place and stores fat
- **Retroperitoneal organs** lie posterior to the peritoneum
- **Intraperitoneal (peritoneal) organs** are surrounded by peritoneum

Splanchnic Circulation
- **Arteries:** Hepatic, splenic, and left gastric from celiac trunk; inferior and superior mesenteric
- **Hepatic portal circulation:** Drains nutrient-rich blood from digestive organs; delivers it to the liver for processing

GI tract regulatory mechanisms
- **Mechanoreceptors and chemoreceptors** - Respond to stretch, changes in osmolarity and pH, and presence of substrate and end products of digestion
  - Initiate reflexes that
    - Activate or inhibit digestive glands
    - Stimulate smooth muscle to mix and move lumen contents
- **Intrinsic and extrinsic controls**
  - **Enteric nerve plexuses** (gut brain) initiate **short reflexes** in response to stimuli in the GI tract
  - **Long reflexes** in response to stimuli inside or outside the GI tract involve CNS centers and autonomic nerves
  - **Hormones** from cells in the stomach and small intestine stimulate target cells in the same or different organs

Parts of the digestive system and their function

Mouth and accessory organs (tongue, teeth, salivary glands)	- **Ingestion**: Intake of food and drinks - **Propulsion**: Swallowing of bolus into pharynx (voluntary buccal phase of deglutition) - **Mechanical digestion**: Chewing (mastication) with help of teeth and tongue - **Chemical digestion**: Salivary amylase breaking down starch
Pharynx	- **Propulsion**: Movement of bolus into esophagus (involuntary pharyngeal-esophageal phase of deglutition)
Esophagus	- **Propulsion**: Movement of bolus to stomach (involuntary pharyngeal-esophageal phase of deglutition)

Stomach	• **Mechanical digestion**: Peristaltic waves churn the bolus until it has creamy consistence • **Propulsion**: Peristaltic waves move chyme into esophagus • **Chemical digestion**: Protein breakdown started by pepsin • **Absorption**: some fat-soluble substances, such as alcohol, aspirin, drugs • **Exocrine-endocrine Gland**: Secretes gastric acid and intrinsic factor into lumen (exocrine function) plus gastrin, histamine, serotonin and somatostatin (endocrine function)
Small intestine and accessory organs (liver, gallbladder, pancreas)	• **Mechanical digestion**: Segmentation assists in the physical breakup of fats and oil • **Propulsion**: Peristaltic waves move the chyme along towards cecum • **Chemical digestion**: Enzymes from pancreas and brush border breakdown all classes of food (proteins, lipids, carbohydrates, nucleic acids); bile needed for emulsification of lipids • **Absorption**: Monosaccharides, amino acids, dipeptides, glycerol, short-chain fatty acids, electrolytes and water absorbed via active or passive transport into capillaries; monoglycerides, long-chain fatty acids and cholesterol packed into chylomicron and transported in lacteals to cistern chyli • **Endocrine gland**: Secretes secretin, cholecystokinin, intestinal gastrin, gastric inhibitory peptide, motilin and vasoactive intestinal peptide
Large intestine	• **Propulsion**: Mass movement propels feces toward rectum and anal canal • **Chemical digestion**: Some remaining food (e.g., cellulose) digested by bacteria • **Absorption**: Electrolytes and water; vitamin K and B if produced by bacteria • **Defecation**: Elimination of feces caused by reflex triggered by rectal distension.

Histology of the Alimentary Canal

Mucosa	• Secretes mucus, digestive enzymes and hormones
	• Absorbs end products of digestion
	• Protects against infectious disease
	• Simple columnar **epithelium** and **mucus-secreting cells**
	• **Lamina propria**: Loose areolar connective tissue
	  • Capillaries for nourishment and absorption
	  • Lymphoid follicles (part of **MALT**)
	• **Muscularis mucosae**: smooth muscle produces local movements of mucosa

Submucosa	• Blood and lymphatic vessels, lymphoid follicles, and submucosal nerve plexus
Muscularis externa	• Responsible for segmentation and peristalsis • **Inner circular** and **outer longitudinal** layers

	• **Myenteric nerve plexus**
	• **Sphincters** in some regions
Serosa	• Visceral peritoneum

Figure 21.1 Gastrointestinal tract and accessory digestive organs

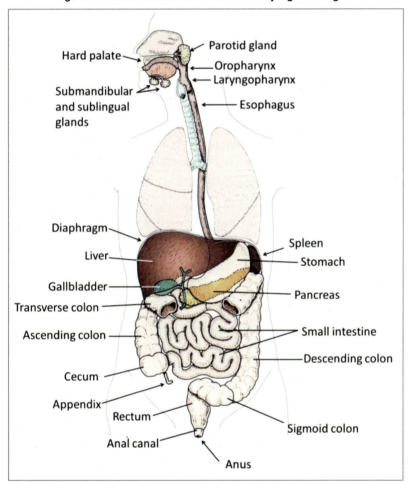

Regulatory Mechanisms

Enteric Nervous System
- Intrinsic nerve supply of the alimentary canal
  - **Submucosal nerve plexus** - Regulates glands and smooth muscle in the mucosa
  - **Myenteric nerve plexus** - Controls GI tract motility: linked to the CNS via afferent visceral fibers
  - **Long ANS fibers** synapse with enteric plexuses
    - **Sympathetic impulses** inhibit secretion and motility
    - **Parasympathetic impulses** stimulate

GI tract reflexes	
Vagovagal reflexes	Stomach/duodenum → brain stem → stomach/duodenum Controls gastric motor and secretory activity
Pain reflexes	Overall inhibition of GI tract
Enterogastric reflex	From duodenum to regulate gastric emptying
Gastroileal reflex	Gastric distention relaxes ileocecal sphincter
Intestino-intestinal reflex	Over-distention or injury of bowel segment causes entire bowel to relax
Gastrocolic reflex	Distention of stomach initiates mass movement
Duodenocolic reflex	Distention of duodenum initiates mass movement
Defecation reflex	Parasympathetic reflex (sacral division) Colon/rectum → spinal cord → colon/rectum Rectal distention initiates defecation

Major hormones of the digestive system

Gastrin	• **Production site:** G cells of gastric glands • **Release stimulus:** Food in stomach (esp. proteins); ACh release by vagus nerve • **Effect(s):** Increased HCl secretion; stimulates gastric emptying; contraction of smooth muscles of small intestine, relaxation of ileocecal sphincter; mass movement in large intestine
Histamine	• **Production site:** Enteroendocrine cells of gastric mucosa • **Release stimulus:** Food in stomach • **Effect(s):** Increased HCl secretion
Serotonin	• **Production site:** Enteroendocrine cells of gastric mucosa • **Release stimulus:** Food in stomach • **Effect(s):** Contraction of gastric smooth muscles
Cholecystokinin [CCK]	• **Production site:** Enteroendocrine cells of duodenal mucosa • **Release stimulus:** Fatty chime; partially digested proteins • **Effect(s):** Increased secretion of bile and enzyme-rich juice; contraction of gallbladder; relaxation of hepatopancreatic sphincter
Secretin	• **Production site:** Enteroendocrine cells of duodenal mucosa • **Release stimulus:** Acidic chyme; partially digested proteins and fats; hypotonic or hypertonic chyme • **Effect(s):** Increased HCl secretion; stimulates gastric emptying; contraction of smooth muscles of small intestine, relaxation of ileocecal sphincter; mass movement in large intestine

Mouth

Oral (buccal) cavity: Bounded by lips, cheeks, palate, and tongue
- **Oral orifice** is the anterior opening
- **Lips and Cheeks** contain orbicularis oris and buccinator muscles
- **Vestibule**: recess internal to lips and cheeks, external to teeth and gums

- **Oral cavity proper** lies within the teeth and gums
- **Digestive Processes:**
  - **Ingestion**
  - **Mechanical digestion**: Mastication is partly voluntary, partly reflexive
  - **Chemical digestion**: Salivary amylase breaks down starch
  - **Propulsion**: Deglutition (swallowing) involves the tongue, soft palate, pharynx, esophagus, and 22 muscle groups
    - **Buccal phase** - Voluntary contraction of the tongue
    - **Pharyngeal-esophageal phase** – Involuntary; control center in the medulla and lower pons

Palate	- **Hard palate**: palatine bones and palatine processes of the maxillae - Slightly corrugated to help create friction against the tongue - **Soft palate**: fold formed mostly of skeletal muscle - Closes off the nasopharynx during swallowing - **Uvula** projects downward from its free edge

Tongue	- **Intrinsic muscles** change the shape of the tongue
	- **Extrinsic muscles** alter the tongue's position
	- **Lingual frenulum**: attachment to the floor of the mouth
	- Surface bears **papillae**
	  - **Filiform** - whitish, give the tongue roughness and provide friction
	  - **Fungiform**, **circumvallate** or **vallate** and **foliate** house taste buds
	- **Terminal sulcus** marks the division between
	  - **Body**: anterior 2/3 residing in the oral cavity
	  - **Root**: posterior 1/3 residing in the oropharynx

Teeth	- Primary and permanent dentitions are formed by age 21
	- 20 **deciduous teeth** erupt (6–24 months of age)
	- 32 **permanent teeth** - all except third molars erupt by the end of adolescence
	  - **Incisors**: Chisel shaped for cutting
	  - **Canines**: Fanglike teeth that tear or pierce
	  - **Premolars (bicuspids) and molars**: Have broad crowns with rounded cusps for grinding or crushing

Salivary Glands	- **Intrinsic (buccal) salivary glands** are scattered in the oral mucosa; continuously keep the mouth moist
	- **Extrinsic salivary glands** produce secretions when
	  - Ingested food stimulates chemoreceptors and mechanoreceptors in the mouth
	  - Nuclei in the brain stem send impulses along **parasympathetic fibers** in cranial nerves VII and IX
	- Strong **sympathetic stimulation** inhibits salivation and results in dry mouth (xerostomia)
	- **Parotid gland** - Anterior to the ear external to the masseter muscle; **parotid duct** opens into the vestibule next to second upper molar
	- **Submandibular gland** - Medial to the body of the mandible; duct

	opens at the base of the lingual frenulum
	• **Sublingual gland** - Anterior to the submandibular gland under the tongue; opens via 10–12 ducts into the floor of the mouth
	• **Saliva** - Cleanses the mouth; moistens and dissolves food chemicals; aids in bolus formation; amylase breaks down starch
	• **Composition**: 97–99.5% water, slightly acidic solution containing
	  • Electrolytes - Na^+, K^+, Cl^-, PO_4^{2-}, HCO_3^-
	  • Salivary amylase
	  • Metabolic wastes - urea and uric acid
	  • Lysozyme, IgA, defensins, and a cyanide compound protect against microorganisms

Pharynx

- Oropharynx and laryngopharynx
- Allow passage of food, fluids, and air
- **Skeletal muscle layers**: inner longitudinal, outer pharyngeal constrictors

Esophagus

- Flat muscular tube from laryngopharynx to stomach
- Pierces diaphragm at esophageal hiatus
- Joins stomach at the **cardiac orifice**
- **Esophageal glands** in submucosa secrete mucus to aid in bolus movement
- **Muscularis**: skeletal superiorly; smooth inferiorly

Figure 21.2 Parts of the stomach

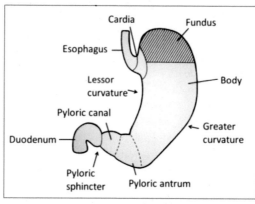

Stomach

Macroscopic Anatomy	• **Cardia**: Surrounds the cardiac orifice • **Fundus**: Dome-shaped region beneath the diaphragm • **Body**: Midportion • **Pyloric region**: antrum, pyloric canal, and pylorus • **Pylorus** is continuous with the duodenum through the pyloric valve (sphincter) • **Greater curvature**: Convex lateral surface

Microscopic Anatomy	• **Lesser curvature**: Concave medial surface • **Muscularis externa** - Three layers of smooth muscle; inner oblique layer allows stomach to churn, mix, move, and physically break down food • **Mucosa** - Layer of mucus traps bicarbonate-rich fluid beneath it • **Gastric pits** lead into **gastric glands**; glands in the fundus and body produce most of the gastric juice

Gastric glands	• **Mucous neck cells** (secrete thin, acidic mucus)
	• **Parietal cells**
	  • **HCl**: → pH 1.5–3.5 denatures protein in food, activates pepsin, and kills many bacteria
	  • **Intrinsic factor**: Glycoprotein required for absorption of vitamin B_{12} in small intestine; lack of intrinsic factor → pernicious anemia
	• **Chief cell**: Inactive enzyme **pepsinogen**
	  • Activated to pepsin by HCl and by pepsin itself (a positive feedback mechanism)
	• **Enteroendocrine cells**: Secrete chemical messengers into the lamina propria
	  • **Paracrines**: Serotonin and histamine
	  • **Hormones**: Somatostatin and gastrin

Mucosal Barrier	• Layer of bicarbonate-rich mucus • **Tight junctions** between epithelial cells • Damaged epithelial cells are quickly replaced by division of stem cells • **Gastritis**: inflammation caused by anything that breaches the mucosal barrier • **Peptic or gastric ulcers**: erosion of the stomach wall; most are caused by *Helicobacter pylori* bacteria

Regulation of Gastric Secretion	• Neural and hormonal mechanisms
	• Stimulatory and inhibitory events occur in three phases:
	  • **Cephalic (reflex) phase**: few minutes prior to food entry
	  • **Gastric phase**: after food enters the stomach; lasts 3–4 hours
	  • **Intestinal phase**: brief stimulatory effect as partially digested food enters the duodenum, followed by inhibitory effects (enterogastric reflex and enterogastrones)

HCl Secretion	• Three chemicals (**ACh, histamine, and gastrin**) stimulate parietal cells through second-messenger systems • All three are necessary for maximum HCl secretion • Antihistamines block H_2 receptors and decrease HCl release
Response to Filling	• Stretches to accommodate incoming food • **Reflex-mediated receptive relaxation** - Coordinated by the swallowing center of the brain stem • **Gastric accommodation** - Plasticity (stress-relaxation response) of smooth muscle
Gastric Con-	• **Peristaltic waves** move toward the pylorus at the rate of 3 per minute

tractile Activity	- **Basic electrical rhythm** (BER) initiated by pacemaker cells (**cells of Cajal**)
- Distension and gastrin increase force of contraction
- Most vigorous near the pylorus
- **Chyme** is either delivered in ~ 30 ml spurts to the duodenum, or forced backward into the stomach
Regulation of Gastric Emptying	- As chyme enters the duodenum
- Receptors respond to stretch and chemical signals
- Enterogastric reflex and enterogastrones inhibit gastric secretion and duodenal filling
- **Carbohydrate-rich chyme** moves quickly through the duodenum
- **Fatty chyme** remains in the duodenum 6 hours or more

Small Intestine

- Major organ of digestion and absorption
- 7-14 feet (2–4 m) long; **from pyloric sphincter to ileocecal valve**
- **Subdivisions**
  - Duodenum
  - Jejunum
  - Ileum

- **Structural Modifications** increase surface area of proximal part for nutrient absorption
  - **Circular folds**: Permanent (~1 cm deep); force chyme to slowly spiral through lumen
  - **Villi**: Motile fingerlike extensions (~1 mm high) of the mucosa; villus epithelium: absorptive cells (**enterocytes**), goblet cells
  - **Microvilli**: Projections (**brush border**) of absorptive cells; bear **brush border enzymes**

- **Intestinal Crypts**
  - **Secretory cells** that produce intestinal juice
  - **Enteroendocrine cells**: Cholecystokinin, secretin and other hormones
  - **Intraepithelial lymphocytes** (IELs): Release cytokines that kill infected cells
  - **Paneth cells**: Secrete antimicrobial agents (defensins and lysozyme)

- **Submucosa**
  - Peyer's patches protect distal part against bacteria
  - **Duodenal (Brunner's) glands** of the duodenum secrete alkaline mucus

---

- **Intestinal Juice** - Secreted in response to distension or irritation of the mucosa
  - **Slightly alkaline** and isotonic with blood plasma
  - Largely water, enzyme-poor, but contains mucus
  - Facilitates transport and absorption of nutrients

- **Requirements for Digestion and Absorption in the Small Intestine**
  - Slow delivery of hypertonic chyme
  - Delivery of bile, enzymes, and bicarbonate from the liver and pancreas
  - Mixing and propulsion

- **Segmentation** - Initiated by intrinsic pacemaker cells
  - Mixes and moves contents slowly and steadily toward the ileocecal valve
  - Intensity is altered by long and short reflexes
  - Wanes in the late intestinal (fasting) phase
- **Peristalsis** - Initiated by **motilin** in the late intestinal phase
  - Each wave starts distal to the previous (the **migrating motility complex**)
  - Meal remnants, bacteria, and debris are moved to the large intestine
  - **Local enteric neurons** coordinate intestinal motility
  - Cholinergic sensory neurons may activate the myenteric plexus
  - Causes contraction of the circular muscle proximally and of longitudinal muscle distally
  - Forces chyme along the tract
- **Ileocecal sphincter** relaxes and admits chyme into the large intestine when
- **Gastroileal reflex** enhances the force of segmentation in the ileum
- **Gastrin** increases the motility of the ileum
- **Ileocecal valve** flaps close when chyme exerts backward pressure

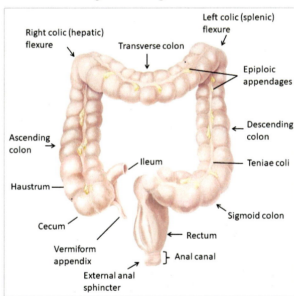

Figure 21.3 Large intestine

Large Intestine

- **Functions of the Large Intestine**
  - Vitamins, water, and electrolytes are reclaimed
  - Major function is propulsion of feces toward the anus
- **Colon is not essential for life**

- Unique features
  - **Teniae coli**: Three bands of longitudinal smooth muscle in the muscularis
  - **Haustra**: Pocketlike sacs caused by the tone of the teniae coli

- **Epiploic appendages**: Fat-filled pouches of visceral peritoneum
- Regions
  - **Cecum** (pouch with attached **vermiform appendix**)
  - **Colon**: Ascending, transverse, descending, and sigmoid colon
  - **Rectum**: Three **rectal valves** stop feces from being passed with gas
  - **Anal canal:** last segment of the large intestine
    - **Internal anal sphincter** - smooth muscle
    - **External anal sphincter** - skeletal muscle
- **Microscopic Anatomy**
  - Abundant **deep crypts** with **goblet cells**
  - **Superficial venous plexuses** of the anal canal form **hemorrhoids** if inflamed
- **Motility of the Large Intestine**
  - **Haustral contractions** - Slow segmenting movements; haustra sequentially contract in response to distension
  - **Gastrocolic reflex** - Initiated by presence of food in the stomach; activates three to four slow powerful peristaltic waves per day in the colon (**mass movements**)
  - **Defecation**
    - Mass movements force feces into rectum → distension initiates spinal **defecation reflex**
    - **Parasympathetic signals** stimulate contraction of the sigmoid colon and rectum → relax the internal anal sphincter
    - **Conscious control allows relaxation of external anal sphincter**
- **Bacterial Flora**
  - Enter from the small intestine or anus
  - Colonize the colon
  - Ferment indigestible carbohydrates
  - Release irritating acids and gases
  - Synthesize B complex vitamins and vitamin K

Accessory Digestive Organs

Liver

- Largest gland in the body
  - Processes bloodborne nutrients
  - Stores fat-soluble vitamins
  - Detoxification
  - Produces bile (~900 ml per day)
- **Four lobes** - right, left, caudate, and quadrate
- **Lesser omentum** anchors liver to stomach
- Hepatic artery and vein at the **porta hepatis**
- **Bile ducts**
  - **Common hepatic duct** leaves the liver
  - **Cystic duct** connects to gallbladder
  - **Bile duct** formed by the union of the above two ducts; bile duct and **main pancreatic duct** join at the **hepatopancreatic ampulla** and enter the duodenum at the **major duodenal papilla**; controlled by the **hepatopancreatic sphincter**

- **Microscopic Anatomy**
  - **Liver lobules** - Hexagonal structural and functional units
  - Filter and process nutrient-rich blood
  - Composed of plates of **hepatocytes** (liver cells)
  - Longitudinal central vein
  - **Portal triad** at each corner of lobule
    - **Bile duct** receives bile from bile canaliculi
    - **Portal arteriole** is a branch of the hepatic artery
    - **Hepatic venule** is a branch of the hepatic portal vein
  - **Liver sinusoids** are leaky capillaries between hepatic plates
    - **Kupffer cells** (hepatic macrophages) in liver sinusoids

- **Bile** - Yellow-green, alkaline solution containing
  - **Bile salts**: cholesterol derivatives that function in fat emulsification and absorption
  - **Bilirubin**: pigment formed from heme
  - **Cholesterol**, neutral fats, phospholipids, and electrolytes
  - **Enterohepatic circulation**: Bile salts → duodenum → reabsorbed from ileum → hepatic portal blood → liver → secreted into bile

- **Gallbladder** - Thin-walled muscular sac on the ventral surface of the liver
  - Stores and concentrates bile by absorbing its water and ions
  - Releases bile via the cystic duct, which flows into the bile duct

- **Bile secretion** is stimulated by
  - Bile salts in enterohepatic circulation
  - **Secretin** from intestinal cells exposed to HCl and fatty chyme
- **Gallbladder contraction** is stimulated by
  - **Cholecystokinin** (CCK) from intestinal cells exposed to proteins and fat in chyme
  - **Vagal stimulation** (minor stimulus)
- CCK also causes the **hepatopancreatic sphincter** to relax

Pancreas

- **Location**: Mostly retroperitoneal, deep to the greater curvature of the stomach
- **Head** is encircled by the duodenum; **tail** abuts the spleen
- **Endocrine function**: Pancreatic islets secrete **insulin** and **glucagon**
- **Exocrine function**: Acini secrete **pancreatic juice**; **zymogen granules** of secretory cells contain digestive enzymes

- **Pancreatic Juice**
  - Watery **alkaline solution** (pH 8) neutralizes chyme
  - Electrolytes (primarily **HCO_3^-**)
  - **Enzymes**
    - Amylase, lipases, nucleases are secreted in active form but require ions or bile for optimal activity
    - Proteases secreted in inactive form; activation in duodenum

- **Regulation of Pancreatic Secretion**
  - **CCK** induces the secretion of enzyme-rich pancreatic juice by acini
  - **Secretin** causes secretion of bicarbonate-rich pancreatic juice by duct cells

> - **Vagal stimulation** also causes release of pancreatic juice (minor stimulus)

Digestion and Absorption

Mechanical Digestion
- Mechanical Digestion **Mouth and accessory organs** (tongue, teeth, salivary glands): Chewing (mastication) with help of teeth and tongue
- **Stomach**: Peristaltic waves churn the bolus until it has creamy consistence
- **Small intestine**: Segmentation assists in the physical breakup of fats and oil into tiny droplets in a process called **emulsification**

Chemical Digestion and Absorption
- **Carbohydrates**
  - **Digestive enzymes:** Salivary amylase, pancreatic amylase, and brush border enzymes (dextrinase, glucoamylase, lactase, maltase, and sucrase)
  - **Absorption**
    - Secondary active transport (cotransport) with Na^+
    - Facilitated diffusion of some monosaccharides
    - Enter the capillary beds in the villi
    - Transported to the liver via the **hepatic portal vein**

- **Proteins**
  - **Enzymes**: Pepsin in the stomach; pancreatic proteases (trypsin, chymotrypsin, and carboxypeptidase), brush border enzymes (aminopeptidases, carboxypeptidases, and dipeptidases)
  - **Absorption** of amino acids is coupled to active transport of Na^+

- **Lipids**
  - Pre-treatment - **emulsification by bile salts**
  - **Enzymes** - pancreatic lipase
  - **Absorption** of **glycerol and short chain fatty acids**: Absorbed into the capillary blood in villi; transported via the hepatic portal vein
  - **Absorption** of **monoglycerides and fatty acids**: Cluster with bile salts and lecithin to form **micelles**; released by micelles to diffuse into epithelial cells; combine with proteins to form **chylomicrons;** enter **lacteals** and are transported to systemic circulation

- **Nucleic Acids**
  - **Enzymes**: Pancreatic ribonuclease and deoxyribonuclease
  - **Absorption**: Active transport; transported to liver via hepatic portal vein

Vitamin Absorption
- In small intestine
  - **Fat-soluble vitamins** (A, D, E, and K) are carried by micelles and then diffuse into absorptive cells
  - **Water-soluble vitamins** (vitamin C and B vitamins) are absorbed by diffusion or by passive or active transporters.
  - **Vitamin B_{12}** binds with intrinsic factor, and is absorbed by endocytosis
- In large intestine
  - **Vitamin K and B vitamins** from bacterial metabolism are absorbed

Electrolyte Absorption - Mostly along the length of small intestine

- Iron and calcium are absorbed in duodenum
- Na^+ is coupled with absorption of glucose and amino acids
- Ionic iron is stored in mucosal cells with ferritin
- K^+ diffuses in response to osmotic gradients
- Ca^{2+} absorption is regulated by vitamin D and parathyroid hormone (PTH)

Water Absorption - 95% is absorbed in the small intestine by osmosis
- Net osmosis occurs whenever a concentration gradient is established by active transport of solutes
- Water uptake is coupled with solute uptake

Digestive enzymes

Enzyme(s)	Origin	Action
Salivary amylase	Salivary glands	Starch -> oligosaccharides and disaccharides
Pancreatic amylase	Exocrine pancreas	Starch -> oligosaccharides and disaccharides
Pepsin	Chief cells of gastric glands; released as inactive pepsinogen; activated by HCl and pepsin	Protein -> large polypeptides
Proteases (trypsin, chymotrypsin, carboxypeptidase)	Exocrine pancreas; all released in inactive form into small intestinal lumen	Large polypeptides -> small peptides
Lipases	Exocrine pancreas	Triglycerides -> glycerol, short-chain fatty acids, long-chain fatty acids, monoglycerides
Ribonuclease and deoxyribonuclease	Exocrine pancreas	Nucleic acids -> pentose sugars, N-containing bases, phosphate ions
Brush border enzymes		
Disaccharidases (dextrinase, glucoamylase, lactase, maltase, sucrose)	Brush border cells in small intestine	Disaccharides -> monosaccharides Lactose -> glucose & galactose Sucrose -> glucose & fructose Maltose -> glucose
Proteases (aminopeptidase, carboxypeptidase, dipeptidase)		Small peptides -> amino acids and some dipeptides and tripeptides
Nucleosidases, phosphatases		Nucleic acids -> pentose sugars, N-containing bases, phosphate ions

Absorption of nutrients

Nutrient(s)	Path of absorption
Glucose, galactose	Active cotransport with Na+ ions -> capillaries -> hepatic portal vein -> liver
Fructose	Facilitated diffusion -> capillaries -> hepatic portal vein -> liver
Amino acids	Active cotransport with Na+ ions -> capillaries -> hepatic portal vein -> liver
Dipeptides and tripeptides	Active cotransport with H+ ions; hydrolyzed to amino acids in epithelial cells -> capillaries -> hepatic portal vein -> liver
Glycerol and short-chain fatty acids	Diffusion into epithelial cells -> capillaries -> hepatic portal vein -> liver
Monoglycerides and fatty acids	Diffusion into epithelial cells; resynthesized to triglycerides; coated with protein to form chylomicrons -> lacteals -> venous system
Cholesterol	Diffusion into epithelial cells; part of chylomicrons -> lacteals -> venous system
Pentose sugars, N-containing bases, phosphate ions	Active transport via membrane carriers -> capillaries -> hepatic portal vein -> liver
Water-soluble vitamins	Diffusion, active or passive processes; vitamin B_{12} needs intrinsic factor -> capillaries -> hepatic portal vein -> liver
Fat-soluble vitamins	Diffusion into epithelial cells; part of chylomicrons -> lacteals -> venous system
Electrolytes	Na^+ and Cl^- active transport; K^+ via facilitated diffusion; Ca^{2+} facilitated diffusion regulated by vitamin D3
Water	Osmosis

Metabolism

Metabolism: biochemical reactions inside cells involving nutrients
- **Anabolism**: synthesis of large molecules from small ones
- **Catabolism**: hydrolysis of complex structures to simpler ones
- **Cellular respiration**: catabolism of food fuels and capture of energy to form ATP in cells
  - Enzymes shift high-energy phosphate groups of ATP to other molecules (phosphorylation)
  - Phosphorylated molecules are activated to perform cellular functions

Stages of Metabolism
- **Digestion, absorption and transport** of nutrients to tissues
- **Cellular processing** (in cytoplasm)
  - Synthesis of lipids, proteins, and glycogen, or
  - Catabolism (glycolysis) into intermediates

A&P Essentials 4th ed.

- **Oxidative (mitochondrial) breakdown** of intermediates into CO2, water, and ATP

Nutrients

Nutrient: a substance in food that promotes normal growth, maintenance, and repair
- **Major nutrients**: Carbohydrates, lipids, and proteins
- **Other nutrients**: Vitamins and minerals (and water)

Catabolic and anabolic pathways of major nutrients

Glucose
- **Energy yield for glucose** and other carbohydrates is **4 kcal per gram**
- **Catabolic pathways**
  - Glycolysis in cytosol
  - Krebs cycle in mitochondria
  - Electron transport chain & oxidative phosphorylation in mitochondria
  - **Glycogenolysis**: Glycogen breakdown in response to low blood glucose
- **Anabolic pathways**
  - **Glycogenesis**: Formation and storage of glycogen in liver and muscle tissue
  - **Gluconeogenesis**: Glucose formation from noncarbohydrate (glycerol and amino acid) molecules; mainly in the liver; protects against damaging effects of hypoglycemia
  - **Lipogenesis**: Triglyceride synthesis and storage via acetyl CoA

Triglycerides
- **Fat catabolism yields** more energy (**9 kcal/g**) than breakdown of carbohydrates or proteins (4 kcal/g)
- **Catabolic pathways**
  - **Glycerol pathway** (Equivalent to $1/2$ glucose): Glycerol is converted to glyceraldehyde phosphate → Krebs cycle Krebs cycle in mitochondria
  - **Fatty acid pathway**: Beta oxidation → 2C fragments → Krebs cycle + reduced coenzymes
  - **Lipolysis**: The reverse of lipogenesis; without oxaloacetic acid acetyl CoA is converted by ketogenesis in the liver into **ketone bodies** (ketones)
- **Anabolic pathways**
  - **Lipogenesis**: Triglyceride synthesis occurs when cellular ATP and glucose levels are high
  - **Synthesis of cholesterol and** transport lipoproteins from acetyl CoA in liver
  - **Synthesis of phospholipids** for cell membranes and myelin

Cholesterol
- **Catabolic pathways**: Not used in catabolic pathways
- **Anabolic pathways**: **Steroid hormone synthesis** in adrenal cortex and gonads (ovaries, testes)

Proteins
- **Energy yield for proteins** is the same as for carbohydrates, i.e., **4 kcal per gram**
- **Catabolic pathways**: Deamination in liver → pyruvic acid → Krebs cycle
  - NH_3 is toxic → combined with CO_2 → urea → kidney → excretion in urine
- **Anabolic pathways**: **Synthesis of structural and functional proteins** depends on complete set of amino acids, essential amino acids must be provided in the diet, non-

essential amino acids can be formed in the body

Catabolic-Anabolic Steady State

Absorptive (fed) state - During and shortly after eating absorption of nutrients is occurring
- **Carbohydrates**
  - Glucose is the major energy fuel
  - Glucose is converted to glycogen or fat
- **Fats**
  - Lipoprotein lipase hydrolyzes lipids of chylomicrons in muscle and fat tissues
  - Most glycerol and fatty acids are converted to triglycerides for storage
  - Triglycerides are used by adipose tissue, liver, and skeletal and cardiac muscle as a primary energy source
- **Proteins**
  - Most amino acids are used in protein synthesis
  - Excess amino acids are deaminated and used for ATP synthesis or stored as fat in the liver
- **Hormonal Control**: Insulin

Postabsorptive (fasting) state - When the GI tract is empty energy sources are supplied by breakdown of reserves
- **Catabolism** of fat, glycogen, and proteins **exceeds anabolism**
  - Goal is to maintain blood glucose between meals
  - Makes glucose available to the blood
  - Promotes use of fats for energy (**glucose sparing**)
- **Sources of Blood Glucose**
  - **Glycogenolysis** in the liver
  - **Glycogenolysis** in skeletal muscle
  - **Lipolysis** in adipose tissues and the liver
  - Glycerol is used for **gluconeogenesis** in the liver
  - **Catabolism of cellular protein** during prolonged fasting
  - Amino acids are deaminated and used for **gluconeogenesis** in the liver and (later) in the kidneys
- **Hormonal Controls**: Glucagon
- **Neural Controls**: In response to low plasma glucose, or during fight-or-flight or exercise, the sympathetic nervous system and epinephrine from the adrenal medulla promote
  - Fat mobilization
  - Glycogenolysis

Comparison of insulin and glucagon	
Insulin	**Glucagon**
• **Release** from pancreatic beta cells is stimulated by	• **Release** from pancreatic alpha cells is stimulated by
• Elevated blood levels of glucose and amino acids	• Declining blood glucose
• GIP and parasympathetic stimulation	• Rising amino acid levels

- **Enhances**
  - Facilitated diffusion of glucose into muscle and adipose cells
  - Glucose oxidation
  - Glycogen and triglyceride formation
  - Active transport of amino acids into tissue cells
  - Protein synthesis

- **Promotes**
  - Glycogenolysis and gluconeogenesis in the liver
  - Lipolysis in adipose tissue
  - Modulation of glucose effects after a high-protein, low-carbohydrate meal
  - Use of fats for energy (**glucose sparing**)

Metabolic Role of the Liver

- Liver cells (hepatocytes) can process nearly every class of nutrient, metabolize alcohol, drugs, hormones, and bilirubin, and produce bile
- Only the liver can deaminate amino acids and create urea from ammonia and carbon dioxide
- Produces most plasma proteins, such as albumin and blood clotting factors
- **Bilirubin formation and** its **excretion** in the bile can be used as a clinical diagnostic tool
- The liver turns unconjugated bilirubin to water-soluble **conjugated bilirubin**.
- Conjugated bilirubin is **secreted** as part of the bile **into the duodenum**. There, ~ 50% is converted by gut bacteria to yellow **urobilinogen**
- Urobilinogen in the feces is oxidized by gut bacteria to brown **stercobilin** that gives feces its color

Figure 21.4 Bilirubin formation and excretion

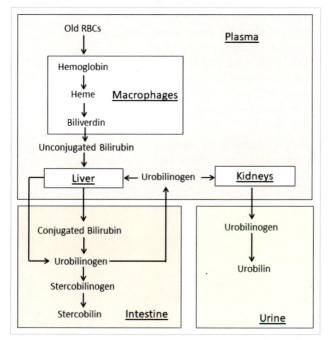

Cholesterol

- Structural basis of bile salts, steroid hormones, and vitamin D
- Major component of plasma membranes
- Makes up part of the hedgehog signaling molecule that directs embryonic development
- Transported in lipoprotein complexes containing triglycerides, phospholipids, cholesterol, and protein

Lipoproteins

- **HDLs (high-density lipoproteins):** The highest protein content; transport excess cholesterol from peripheral tissues to the liver to be broken down and secreted into bile; also provide cholesterol to steroid-producing organs
- **LDLs (low-density lipoproteins):** Cholesterol-rich; transport cholesterol to peripheral tissues for membranes, storage, or hormone synthesis
- **VLDLs (very low density lipoproteins):** Mostly triglycerides; transport triglycerides to peripheral tissues (mostly adipose)
- **Chylomicrons:** Mostly triglycerides, depending on nutrition
  - **High levels of HDL** are thought to protect against heart attack
  - **High levels of LDL**, especially lipoprotein (a) increase the risk of heart attack

Plasma Cholesterol Levels

- The liver produces cholesterol
  - At a basal level regardless of dietary cholesterol intake
  - In response to saturated fatty acids
- **Saturated fatty acids:** Stimulate liver synthesis of cholesterol; inhibit cholesterol excretion from the body
- **Unsaturated fatty acids:** Enhance excretion of cholesterol
- **Trans fats:** Increase LDLs and reduce HDLs
- **Unsaturated omega-3 fatty acids** (found in cold-water fish): Lower the proportions of saturated fats and cholesterol
  - Have antiarrhythmic effects on the heart
  - Help prevent spontaneous clotting
  - Lower blood pressure

Non-Dietary Factors Affecting Cholesterol

- Stress, cigarette smoking, and coffee lower HDL levels
- Aerobic exercise and estrogen increase HDL levels and decrease LDL levels
- Body shape
  - "**Apple**": Fat carried on the upper body is correlated with high cholesterol and LDL levels
  - "**Pear**": Fat carried on the hips and thighs is correlated with lower cholesterol and LDL levels

Chapter 22 Urinary System

Urinary System Organs

- **Kidneys** - major excretory organs
  - Removal of toxins, metabolic wastes, and excess ions from the blood
  - Regulation of blood volume, chemical composition, and pH
  - Gluconeogenesis during prolonged fasting
  - Endocrine functions
    - **Renin**: regulation of blood pressure and kidney function
    - **Erythropoietin**: regulation of RBC production
    - Activation of **vitamin D**
- **Urinary bladder** - temporary storage reservoir for urine
- **Ureters** - transport of urine from the kidneys to the bladder
- **Urethra** – transport of urine out of the body

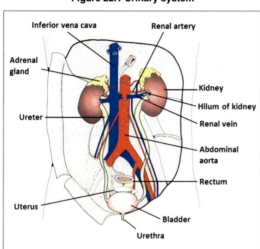

Figure 22.1 Urinary system

Kidney Anatomy

- Bean-shaped retroperitoneal organs; right kidney lower than left
- Convex lateral surface, concave medial surface
- **Renal hilum** leads to the **renal sinus** where ureters, renal blood vessels, lymphatics, and nerves enter and exit
- Layers of supportive tissue
  - **Renal fascia**: The anchoring outer layer of dense fibrous connective tissue
  - **Perirenal fat capsule**: A fatty cushion
  - **Fibrous capsule**: Surrounds the kidney itself
- **Renal cortex**: A granular superficial region
- **Renal medulla**: The cone-shaped medullary (renal) **pyramids** separated by **renal columns**
  - **Papilla**: Tip of pyramid; releases urine into minor calyx

- **Renal pelvis**: The funnel-shaped tube within the renal sinus
- **Major calyces**: The branching channels of the renal pelvis that collect urine from **minor calyces**
- Empty urine into the **renal pelvis**
- Urine flows from the pelvis to **ureter**
- **Renal arteries** deliver ~ $1/4$ (1200 ml) of cardiac output to the kidneys each minute

Nephron and collecting ducts

Nephron - Structural and functional units that form urine; ~1 million per kidney
- **Cortical nephrons** - 85% of nephrons; almost entirely in the cortex
- **Juxtamedullary nephrons** - Long loops of Henle deeply invade the medulla; important in the production of concentrated urine
- **Glomerulus**: a tuft of capillaries
- **Renal tubule**: begins as cup-shaped glomerular (Bowman's) capsule surrounding the glomerulus
- **Renal corpuscle**: Glomerulus + its glomerular capsule; fenestrated glomerular endothelium allows filtrate to pass from plasma into the glomerular capsule

Renal Tubule
- **Glomerular (Bowman's) capsule**
  - **Parietal layer**: simple squamous epithelium
  - **Visceral layer**: branching epithelial **podocytes**
    - Extensions terminate in **foot processes** that cling to basement membrane
    - **Filtration slits** allow filtrate to pass into the capsular space
- **Proximal convoluted tubule** (PCT) - Functions in reabsorption and secretion; confined to the cortex
- **Loop of Henle** with descending and ascending limbs
  - **Thin segment** usually in descending limb; freely permeable to water
  - **Thick segment** of ascending limb
- **Distal convoluted tubule** (DCT) - Functions more in secretion than reabsorption; confined to the cortex

Collecting Ducts - Receive filtrate from many nephrons
- Fuse together to deliver urine through papillae into minor calyces
  - **Intercalated cells**: Function in maintaining the acid-base balance of the body
  - **Principal cells**: Help maintain the body's water and salt balance

Nephron Capillary Beds
- **Glomerulus:** Afferent arteriole → glomerulus → efferent arteriole
  - Blood pressure is high because
    - Afferent arterioles are smaller in diameter than efferent arterioles
    - Arterioles are high-resistance vessels
- **Peritubular capillaries:** Low-pressure, porous capillaries adapted for absorption
  - Arise from efferent arterioles; cling to adjacent renal tubules in cortex; empty into venules
- **Vasa recta:** Long vessels parallel to long loops of Henle
  - Arise from efferent arterioles of juxtamedullary nephrons
  - Function information of concentrated urine

- **High resistance in afferent and efferent arterioles** causes blood pressure to decline from ~95 mm Hg to ~8 mm Hg in kidneys
- **Resistance in afferent arterioles** protects glomeruli from fluctuations in systemic blood pressure
- **Resistance in efferent arterioles** reinforces high glomerular pressure and reduces hydrostatic pressure in peritubular capillaries

Figure 22.2 Nephron and collecting duct

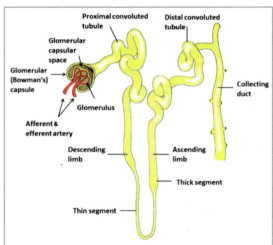

Figure 22.3 Renal corpuscle

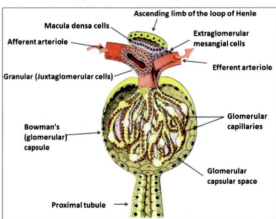

Juxtaglomerular Apparatus (JGA)

- Important in regulation of filtrate formation and blood pressure
- **Granular cells** (juxtaglomerular, or JG cells) - Enlarged, smooth muscle cells of arteriole; secretory granules contain **renin**; mechanoreceptors that sense blood pressure
- **Macula densa** - Tall, closely packed cells of the ascending limb; **chemoreceptors** that sense NaCl content of filtrate

- **Extraglomerular mesangial cells** - Interconnected with gap junctions; may pass signals between macula densa and granular cells

Filtration Membrane

- Porous membrane separating blood and capsular space
  - **Fenestrated endothelium** of the glomerular capillaries
  - **Visceral membrane** of the glomerular capsule (podocytes with foot processes and filtration slits)
  - Gel-like **basement membrane** allows passage of water and solutes smaller than most plasma proteins
  - Fenestrations prevent filtration of blood cells
  - Negatively charged basement membrane repels large anions such as plasma proteins
  - Slit diaphragms also help to repel macromolecules
- **Glomerular mesangial cells** - Engulf and degrade macromolecules
  - Can contract to change the total surface area available for filtration

Ureters

- Convey urine from kidneys to bladder
- Enter the base of the bladder through the posterior wall
- As bladder pressure increases, distal ends of the ureters close, preventing backflow of urine
- **Smooth muscle muscularis**; contracts in response to stretch

Urinary Bladder

- Muscular sac for temporary storage of urine
- Retroperitoneal, on pelvic floor posterior to pubic symphysis
- **Males** - prostate gland surrounds the neck inferiorly
- **Females** - anterior to the vagina and uterus
- **Trigone**: Smooth triangular area outlined by the openings for the ureters and the urethra; infections tend to persist in this region
- Layers of the **bladder wall**
  - Transitional epithelial mucosa
  - Thick detrusor muscle (three layers of smooth muscle)
  - Fibrous adventitia (peritoneum on superior surface only)
- Collapses when empty; **rugae appear**
- Expands and rises superiorly during filling without significant rise in internal pressure

Urethra

- Muscular tube
  - **Internal urethral sphincter** - Involuntary (smooth muscle) at bladder-urethra junction; contracts to open
  - **External urethral sphincter** - Voluntary (skeletal) muscle surrounding the urethra as it passes through the pelvic floor
- **Female urethra** (1-1.5 inches): Tightly bound to the anterior vaginal wall
  - **External urethral orifice** is anterior to the vaginal opening, posterior to the clitoris

- **Male urethra**: Carries semen and urine
  - **Prostatic urethra** (1 inch) - within prostate gland
  - **Membranous urethra** (.8 inch) - passes through the urogenital diaphragm
  - **Spongy urethra** (6 inches) - passes through the penis and opens via the external urethral orifice

Micturition

- Urination or voiding
- Three simultaneous events
  - **Contraction of detrusor muscle** by ANS
  - **Opening of internal urethral sphincter** by ANS
  - **Opening of external urethral sphincter** by somatic nervous system
- **Reflexive urination** (urination in infants)
  - Distension of bladder activates stretch receptors
  - Excitation of parasympathetic neurons in reflex center in sacral region of spinal cord
  - Contraction of the detrusor muscle
  - Contraction (opening) of internal sphincter
  - Inhibition of somatic pathways to external sphincter, allowing its relaxation (opening)

Renal Physiology

- The kidneys filter the body's entire plasma volume 60 times each day = 180 l of filtrate
  - **Glomerular filtration** → Filtrate (blood plasma minus proteins)
  - **Tubular reabsorption** - Returns all glucose and amino acids, 99% of water, salt, and other components to the blood
  - **Tubular secretion** - Reverse of reabsorption: selective addition to urine
  - **Urine**: <1% of total filtrate; contains metabolic wastes and unneeded substances

Glomerular Filtration - Passive mechanical process driven by hydrostatic pressure
- **Glomerular blood pressure** is higher (**55 mm Hg**) than other capillaries (35 mm Hg)
  - Molecules >5 nm are not filtered (e.g., plasma proteins) and function to maintain colloid osmotic pressure of the blood
- **Net Filtration Pressure (NFP)** - **The pressure responsible for filtrate formation** (10 mm Hg); difference between glomerular hydrostatic pressure and the sum of colloid osmotic pressure of glomerular blood and capsular hydrostatic pressure

Glomerular Filtration Rate (GFR) - Volume of filtrate formed per minute by the kidneys (120–125 ml/min); directly proportional to
- Total surface area available for filtration
- Filtration membrane permeability
- Net filtration pressure
- GFR is tightly controlled by two types of mechanisms
  - **Intrinsic controls** (renal autoregulation): Act locally within the kidney; maintain a nearly constant GFR when MAP is in the range of 80–180 mm Hg
    - **Myogenic Mechanism** - Helps maintain normal GFR
      - ↑ BP → constriction of afferent arterioles; protects glomeruli from damaging high BP
      - ↓ BP → dilation of afferent arterioles
    - **Tuboglomerular Feedback Mechanism** senses changes in the JGA

- ↑GFR →flow rate increases in the tubule → filtrate NaCl concentration ↑ because of insufficient time for reabsorption
- Macula densa cells respond by releasing a vasoconstricting chemical that acts on the afferent arteriole → ↓ GFR
- The opposite occurs if ↓GFR.
- **Extrinsic controls**: Nervous and endocrine mechanisms that maintain blood pressure, but affect kidney function
  - Under normal conditions at rest renal blood vessels are dilated, renal autoregulation mechanisms prevail
  - Under extreme stress **norepinephrine** (released by sympathetic nervous system) and **epinephrine** (released by adrenal medulla) cause constriction of afferent arterioles, inhibiting filtration and triggering the release of renin

Renin-Angiotensin Mechanism
- **Triggers for renin release**
  - Reduced stretch of granular cells (MAP below 80 mm Hg)
  - Stimulation of the granular cells by activated macula densa cells
  - Direct stimulation of granular cells via β_1-adrenergic receptors by renal nerves
- **Angiotensin converting hormone** (ACE) leads to formation of **angiotensin II**
- **Angiotensin II**
  - Constricts arteriolar smooth muscle, causing MAP to rise
  - Stimulates the reabsorption of Na^+
  - Triggers adrenal cortex to release aldosterone
  - Stimulates the hypothalamus to release ADH and activates the thirst center
  - Constricts efferent arterioles, decreasing peritubular capillary hydrostatic pressure and increasing fluid reabsorption
  - Causes glomerular mesangial cells to contract, decreasing the surface area available for filtration

Tubular Reabsorption
- All organic nutrients are reabsorbed
- Water and ion reabsorption are hormonally regulated
- Includes active and passive process
- **Transcellular route** - Luminal and basolateral membranes of tubule cells, endothelium of peritubular capillaries
- **Paracellular route** - Limited to water movement and reabsorption of Ca^{2+}, Mg^{2+}, K^+, and some Na^+ in the PCT where tight junctions are leaky
- **Sodium Reabsorption** (most abundant cation in filtrate)
  - **Primary active transport** out of the tubule cell by Na^+-K^+ ATPase in the basolateral membrane; Na^+ passes in through the luminal membrane by secondary active transport or facilitated diffusion mechanisms; promotes bulk flow of water and solutes (including Na^+)
- **Reabsorption of Nutrients, Water, and Ions**
  - Na+ reabsorption provides the energy and the means for reabsorbing most other substances
  - Organic nutrients are reabsorbed by **secondary active transport**
    - **Transport maximum** (Tm) reflects the number of carriers in the renal tubules available; when the carriers are saturated, excess of that substance is excreted
  - **Water** is reabsorbed by osmosis (obligatory water reabsorption), aided by water-

filled pores called **aquaporins**
- **Cations** and **fat-soluble substances** follow by diffusion

Reabsorptive Capabilities of Renal Tubules and Collecting Ducts
- **PCT**: Site of most reabsorption; 65% of Na^+ and water; all nutrients; ions; small proteins
- **Loop of Henle**: Descending limb: H_2O; Ascending limb: Na^+, K^+, Cl^-
- **DCT and collecting duct**: Reabsorption is hormonally regulated; Ca^{2+} (PTH); water (ADH); Na^+ (aldosterone and ANP)

Tubular Secretion
- Disposes of substances that are bound to plasma proteins
- Eliminates undesirable substances that have been passively reabsorbed (e.g., urea)
- Rids the body of excess K^+
- Controls blood pH by altering amounts of H^+ or HCO_3^- in urine

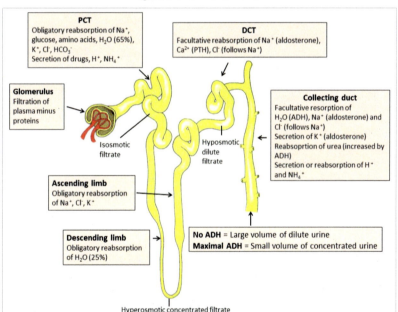

Figure 22.4 Urine formation

Regulation of Urine Concentration and Volume
- **Osmolality**: Number of solute particles in 1 kg of H_2O
  - Osmolality of body fluids expressed in **milliosmols** (mOsm)
  - The **kidneys maintain osmolality of plasma at ~300 mOsm**, using countercurrent mechanisms
- **Countercurrent mechanism** occurs when fluid flows in opposite directions in two adjacent segments of the same tube
  - Filtrate flow in the **loop of Henle** (**countercurrent multiplier**)
    - **Descending limb** - Freely permeable to H_2O; filtrate osmolality increases to ~1200 mOsm

- **Ascending limb** - Impermeable to H_2O; selectively permeable to solutes; Na^+ and Cl^- passively reabsorbed in the thin segment, actively reabsorbed in the thick segment; filtrate osmolality decreases to 100 mOsm
- Blood flow in the vasa recta (**countercurrent exchanger**) maintains the osmotic gradient
- Establishes and maintains an osmotic gradient (300 mOsm to 1200 mOsm) from renal cortex through the medulla that allows the kidneys to vary urine concentration
- **Formation of Dilute Urine**
  - Filtrate is diluted in the ascending loop of Henle
  - In the **absence of ADH**, dilute filtrate continues into the renal pelvis as dilute urine
  - Na^+ and other ions may be selectively removed in the DCT and collecting duct, decreasing osmolality to as low as 50 mOsm
- **Formation of Concentrated Urine**
  - Depends on the medullary osmotic gradient and ADH
  - **ADH triggers reabsorption of H_2O** in the collecting ducts
  - **Facultative water reabsorption** occurs **in the presence of ADH** so that 99% of H_2O in filtrate is reabsorbed

---

Diuretics – Substances that enhance the urinary output
- **Osmotic diuretics**: substances not reabsorbed, (e.g., glucose in a diabetes)
- **ADH inhibitors** such as alcohol
- Substances that inhibit Na^+ reabsorption and obligatory H_2O reabsorption such as **caffeine** and many drugs

---

Renal Clearance - Volume of plasma cleared of a particular substance in a given time
- For any substance freely filtered and neither reabsorbed nor secreted by the kidneys (e.g., inulin), **RC = GFR = 125 ml/min**
  - If RC < 125 ml/min, the substance is reabsorbed
  - If RC = 0, the substance is completely reabsorbed
  - If RC > 125 ml/min, the substance is secreted (most drug metabolites)

Characteristics of Urine

Color and transparency	• Clear, pale to deep yellow (due to urochrome) • Drugs, vitamin supplements, and diet can alter the color • Cloudy urine may indicate a urinary tract infection
Odor	• Slightly aromatic when fresh • Develops ammonia odor upon standing • May be altered by some drugs and vegetables (e.g., asparagus)
pH	• Slightly acidic (~pH 6, with a range of 4.5 to 8.0) • Diet, prolonged vomiting, or urinary tract infections may alter pH
Specific gravity	• 1.001 to 1.035, dependent on solute concentration
Chemical Composition	• 95% water and 5% solutes • **Nitrogenous wastes**: urea, uric acid, and creatinine • Na^+, K^+, PO_4^{3-}, SO_4^{2-}, Ca^{2+}, Mg^{2+} and HCO_3^- • Abnormally high concentrations of any constituent may indicate pathology

Chapter 23 Fluid, Electrolyte, and Acid-Base Balance

Body Water Content

- **Infants**: 73% or more water (low body fat, low bone mass)
- **Adult males**: ~60% water
- **Adult females**: ~50% water (higher fat content, less skeletal muscle mass)
  - Water content declines to ~45% in old age

Composition of Body Fluids

- **Water**: universal solvent
- **Solutes**: nonelectrolytes and electrolytes
  - **Nonelectrolytes** - Do not dissociate in water; most are organic, e.g., glucose, lipids, creatinine, and urea
  - **Electrolytes** - Dissociate into ions in water; e.g., inorganic salts, all acids and bases, some proteins
    - Most abundant solutes, have greater osmotic power than nonelectrolytes, so may contribute to fluid shifts
    - Determine the chemical and physical reactions of fluids

Electrolyte Concentration

- Expressed in **milliequivalents per liter** (mEq/L), a measure of the number of electrical charges per liter of solution
- For **single charged ions** (e.g. Na^+), 1 mEq = 1 mOsm
- For **bivalent ions** (e.g. Ca^{2+}), 1 mEq = 1/2 mOsm

Extracellular and Intracellular Fluids

- Each fluid compartment has a distinctive pattern of electrolytes
- **ECF**: All similar, except higher protein content of plasma; **major cation**: Na^+; **major anion**: Cl^-
- **ICF**: Low Na^+ and Cl^-; **major cation**: K^+; **major anion**: HPO_4^{2-}
- Proteins, phospholipids, cholesterol, and neutral fats make up the bulk of **dissolved solutes**

Fluid Movement among Compartments is regulated by osmotic and hydrostatic pressures

- **Water moves freely by osmosis**; osmolalities of all body fluids are almost always equal; two-way osmotic flow is substantial
- **Ion fluxes** require active transport or channels
- **Change in solute concentration of any compartment leads to net water flow**

Water Balance and ECF Osmolality

Water intake: beverages, food, and metabolic water
- **Regulation: Thirst mechanism is the driving force for water intake**
- The **hypothalamic thirst center** osmoreceptors are stimulated by
  - ↑ Plasma osmolality of 2–3%
  - Angiotensin II or baroreceptor input
  - Dry mouth
  - Substantial decrease in blood volume or pressure
- Drinking water creates inhibition of the thirst center; inhibitory feedback signals include

- Relief of dry mouth
- Activation of stomach and intestinal stretch receptors

Water output: urine, insensible water loss (skin and lungs), perspiration, and feces
- **Obligatory water losses**: Insensible water loss: from lungs and skin
  - Feces
- **Minimum daily sensible water loss of 500 ml in urine** to excrete wastes
- Body water and Na^+ content are regulated in tandem by mechanisms that maintain cardiovascular function and blood pressure
- **Influence of ADH**: Water reabsorption in collecting ducts is proportional to ADH release
  - ↓ ADH → dilute urine and ↓ volume of body fluids
  - ↑ ADH → concentrated urine
- **Hypothalamic osmoreceptors** trigger or inhibit ADH release
- Other factors may trigger ADH release via large changes in blood volume or pressure, e.g., fever, sweating, vomiting, or diarrhea; blood loss; and traumatic burns

Table 23.1 Average daily water balance

Intake		Output	
Source	Amount/%	Loss	Amount/%
Beverages	1500 ml/60%	Urine	1500 ml/60%
Food	750 ml/30%	Insensible loss via skin/lungs	700 ml/28%
Metabolism	250 ml/10%	Sensible loss via sweat	200 ml/8%
		Feces	100 ml/4%
total	2500 ml		2500 ml

Disorders of Water Balance

Dehydration - Negative fluid balance
- **ECF water loss** due to: hemorrhage, severe burns, prolonged vomiting or diarrhea, profuse sweating, water deprivation, diuretic abuse
- **Signs and symptoms**: thirst, dry flushed skin, oliguria
  - May lead to weight loss, fever, mental confusion, hypovolemic shock, and loss of electrolytes

Hypotonic Hydration - Cellular overhydration, or water intoxication
- Occurs with renal insufficiency or rapid excess water ingestion
- ECF is diluted → hyponatremia → net osmosis into tissue cells → swelling of cells → severe metabolic disturbances (nausea, vomiting, muscular cramping, cerebral edema) → possible death

Edema - Atypical accumulation of IF fluid → tissue swelling
- Due to anything that increases flow of fluid out of the blood or hinders its return, e.g., ↑ blood pressure, ↑ capillary permeability, congestive heart failure, ↑ blood volume
- Hindered fluid return occurs with an imbalance in colloid osmotic pressures, e.g.,

hypoproteinemia (↓ plasma proteins)
- Blocked (or surgically removed) **lymph vessels**

Electrolyte Balance

Electrolytes are solutes that dissociate into ions in water, for example, salts, acids, and bases

Electrolyte balance usually refers only to salt balance

Sodium - Most abundant cation in the ECF; Na salts in the ECF contribute 280 mOsm of the total 300 mOsm ECF solute concentration
- Na^+ content may change but ECF Na^+ concentration remains stable due to
- Na^+-water balance is linked to blood pressure and blood volume control mechanisms

- **Aldosterone** → active reabsorption of Na^+ remaining after obligatory resorption
  - Water follows Na^+ if ADH is present
  - **Renin-angiotensin mechanism** is the main trigger for aldosterone release
    - Granular cells of JGA secrete renin in response to
      - Sympathetic nervous system stimulation
      - ↓ Filtrate osmolality
      - ↓ Stretch (due to ↓ blood pressure)
    - Renin catalyzes the production of angiotensin II, which prompts aldosterone release from the adrenal cortex
  - Aldosterone release is also triggered by elevated K^+ levels in the ECF
  - **Aldosterone brings about its effects slowly** (hours to days)
- **ANP** - Released by atrial cells in response to stretch (↑ blood pressure)
  - Decreases blood pressure and blood volume:
    - ↓ ADH, renin and aldosterone production
    - ↑ Excretion of Na^+ and water
  - Promotes vasodilation directly and also by decreasing production of angiotensin II
- **Estrogens**: ↑ NaCl reabsorption (like aldosterone) → H_2O retention during menstrual cycles and pregnancy
- **Progesterone**: ↓ Na^+ reabsorption (blocks aldosterone); promotes Na^+ and H_2O loss
- **Glucocorticoids**: ↑ Na^+ reabsorption and promote edema
- **Cardiovascular System Baroreceptors** alert the brain of increases in blood volume and pressure
  - Sympathetic nervous system impulses to the kidneys decline
  - Afferent arterioles dilate
  - GFR increases
  - Na^+ and water output increase

Potassium Balance

Potassium - Affects RMP in neurons and muscle cells (especially cardiac muscle)
- **Hyperkalemia**: ↑ ECF $[K^+]$ → ↓RMP → depolarization → reduced excitability
- **Hypokalemia** ↓ ECF $[K^+]$ → hyperpolarization and nonresponsiveness
- H^+ shift in and out of cells; leads to shifts in K^+ in the opposite direction to maintain cation balance; interferes with activity of excitable cells

- **K^+ balance** is controlled in the cortical collecting ducts by changing the amount of potassium secreted into filtrate; High K^+ content of ECF favors secretion of K^+; low K^+ levels cells reabsorb some K^+ left in the filtrate
- **Aldosterone** stimulates K^+ secretion (and Na^+ reabsorption) by principal cells
  - Increased K^+ in the adrenal cortex → release of aldosterone → potassium secretion

Calcium Balance

- **Hypocalcemia** → ↑ excitability and muscle tetany
- **Hypercalcemia** → Inhibits neurons and muscle cells, may cause heart arrhythmias
- Calcium balance is controlled by **parathyroid hormone** (PTH) and **calcitonin**
- **PTH** promotes increase in calcium levels by targeting bones, kidneys, and small intestine (indirectly through vitamin D)
- Calcium reabsorption and phosphate excretion go hand in hand
  - Normally 75% of filtered phosphates are actively reabsorbed in the PCT
  - PTH inhibits this by decreasing the T_m

Acid-Base Balance

- Normal **pH of arterial blood 7.4**
  - **Alkalosis**: pH >7.45
  - **Acidosis**: pH < 7.35
- Most H^+ is produced by metabolism, e.g., lactic acid from anaerobic respiration of glucose, fatty acids and ketone bodies from fat metabolism, H^+ liberated when CO_2 is converted to HCO_3^- in blood
- Concentration of hydrogen ions is regulated sequentially by
  - **Chemical buffer systems**: rapid; first line of defense
  - **Brain stem respiratory centers**: act within 1–3 min
  - **Renal mechanisms**: most potent, but require hours to days to effect pH changes
- **Acid-Base Balance**
  - **Chemical buffers** cannot eliminate excess acids or bases from the body
  - **Lungs eliminate volatile carbonic acid** by eliminating CO_2
  - **Kidneys eliminate other fixed metabolic acids** (phosphoric, uric, and lactic acids and ketones) and prevent metabolic acidosis

Chemical Buffer Systems: One or more compounds that act to resist pH changes when strong acid or base is added
- **Bicarbonate Buffer System**: Mixture of H_2CO_3 (weak acid) and salts of HCO_3^- (e.g., $NaHCO_3$, a weak base); buffers ICF and ECF; **the only important ECF buffer**
  - If strong acid is added HCO_3^- ties up H^+ and forms H_2CO_3 → pH decreases only slightly, unless all available HCO_3^- (**alkaline reserve**) is used up
  - If strong base is added it causes H_2CO_3 to dissociate and donate H^+ → H^+ ties up the base (e.g. OH^-) → pH rises only slightly
- **Phosphate Buffer System**
  - Action is nearly identical to the bicarbonate buffer
  - **Effective buffer in urine and ICF**, where phosphate concentrations are high
- **Protein Buffer System**
  - Protein molecules are amphoteric
    - When pH rises, organic acid or carboxyl (COOH) groups release H^+

- When pH falls, NH_2 groups bind H^+
- **Intracellular proteins are the most plentiful and powerful buffers**; plasma proteins also important

Physiological Buffer Systems
- Act more slowly than chemical buffer systems
- Have more capacity than chemical buffer systems
- **Respiratory Regulation of H^+**
  - Respiratory system eliminates CO_2
  - A reversible equilibrium exists in the blood: $CO_2 + H_2O \leftrightarrow H_2CO_3 \leftrightarrow H^+ + HCO_3^-$
  - During CO_2 unloading the reaction shifts to the left (and H^+ is incorporated into H_2O)
  - During CO_2 loading the reaction shifts to the right (and H^+ is buffered by proteins)
  - **Hypercapnia** activates medullary chemoreceptors, rising plasma H^+ activates peripheral chemoreceptors → more CO_2 is removed from the blood → H^+ concentration is reduced
  - Respiratory system impairment causes acid-base imbalances
    - **Hypoventilation** → respiratory acidosis
    - **Hyperventilation** → respiratory alkalosis
- **Renal Mechanisms of Acid-Base Balance**
  - Most important renal mechanisms
    - Secretion of H^+
    - Conserving (reabsorbing) or generating new HCO_3^-
    - Excreting HCO_3^-
  - Generating or reabsorbing one HCO_3^- is the same as losing one H^+
  - Excreting one HCO_3^- is the same as gaining one H^+

Abnormalities of Acid-Base Balance

Respiratory Acidosis and Alkalosis
- The most important indicator of adequacy of respiratory function is P_{CO_2} level (normally 35–45 mm Hg)
- P_{CO_2} above 45 mm Hg → respiratory acidosis
  - Most common cause of acid-base imbalances
  - Due to decrease in ventilation or gas exchange
  - Characterized by falling blood pH and rising P_{CO_2}
- P_{CO_2} below 35 mm Hg → respiratory alkalosis
  - A common result of hyperventilation due to stress or pain

- **Metabolic Acidosis and Alkalosis** - Any pH imbalance not caused by abnormal blood CO_2 levels; Indicated by abnormal HCO_3^- levels
  - Causes of **metabolic acidosis**
    - Ingestion of too much alcohol (→ acetic acid)
    - Excessive loss of HCO_3^- (e.g., persistent diarrhea)
    - Accumulation of lactic acid, shock, ketosis in diabetic crisis, starvation, and kidney failure
  - **Metabolic alkalosis** is much less common than metabolic acidosis; indicated by rising blood pH and HCO_3^-
    - Caused by vomiting of the acid contents of the stomach or by intake of excess

base (e.g., antacids)

Determination of acidosis and alkalosis

Basic facts	• Normal blood pH 7.35-7.45 • Normal pCO_2 35-45 mm Hg • If pH changes are caused by an **elevated or reduced pCO_2** they are called **respiratory** acidosis or alkalosis • **If the pCO_2 is within the normal range** pH changes are **called** metabolic **regardless of the underlying cause**
Step 1: Look at pH	• pH < 7.35 = **Acidosis** • pH > 7.45 = **Alkalosis**
Step 2: Respiratory or metabolic acidosis?	• pH < 7.35 and pCO_2 > 45 = **Respiratory Acidosis** • pH < 7.35 and pCO_2 35-45 = **Metabolic Acidosis**
Step 3: Respiratory or metabolic alkalosis?	• pH > 7.45 and pCO_2 <35 = **Respiratory Alkalosis** • pH > 7.45 and pCO_2 35-45 = **Metabolic Alkalosis**

Effects of Acidosis and Alkalosis

- Blood pH below 7 → depression of CNS → coma → death
- Blood pH above 7.8 → excitation of nervous system → muscle tetanus, extreme nervousness, convulsions, respiratory arrest

Respiratory and Renal Compensations

- If acid-base imbalance is due to malfunction of a physiological buffer system, the other one compensates
  - Respiratory system attempts to correct metabolic acid-base imbalances
  - Kidneys attempt to correct respiratory acid-base imbalances
- **Respiratory Compensation**
  - In **metabolic acidosis** high H^+ levels stimulate the respiratory centers → rate and depth of breathing are elevated
    - As CO_2 is eliminated by the respiratory system, P_{CO2} falls below normal
  - Respiratory compensation for **metabolic alkalosis** is revealed by slow, shallow breathing → CO_2 accumulation in the blood
- **Renal Compensation**
  - Hypoventilation causes elevated P_{CO2} (**respiratory acidosis**)
    - Renal compensation is indicated by high HCO_3^- levels
  - **Respiratory alkalosis** exhibits low P_{CO2} and high pH
    - Renal compensation is indicated by decreasing HCO_3^- levels

Chapter 24 Reproductive System and Pregnancy

Overview

- **Primary sex organs** (gonads): **testes and ovaries**
  - Produce sex cells (gametes)
  - Secrete steroid **sex hormones**
    - **Androgens** (males)
    - **Estrogens and progesterone** (females)
  - Play roles in
    - Development and function of the reproductive organs
    - Sexual behavior and drives
    - Growth and development of many other organs and tissues
- **Accessory reproductive organs**: ducts, glands, and external genitalia
- **Gametogenesis** or the **formation of sex cells** (gametes) is a complex process
- Gametogenesis involves two different types of cell division, **mitotic division** that yields genetically identical daughter cells, and **meiosis** that leads to cells with a haploid chromosome set
- Sex cells are haploid, i.e., they have one set of 23 chromosomes only

Male Reproductive System

Testes (testicles)
- Each is surrounded by two tunics
  - **Tunica vaginalis**, derived from peritoneum
  - **Tunica albuginea**, the fibrous capsule
- **Septa** divide the testis into 250–300 **lobules**, each containing 1–4 seminiferous tubules (site of sperm production)
  - Sperm are conveyed through seminiferous tubules → tubulus rectus → rete testis → efferent ductules → epididymis
- **Blood supply** comes from the testicular arteries and testicular veins
- **Spermatic cord** encloses nerve fibers, blood vessels, and lymphatics that supply the testes
- **Interstitial (Leydig) cells** outside the seminiferous tubules **produce androgens**

Scrotum
- Sac of skin and superficial fascia
- Hangs outside the abdominopelvic cavity
- Contains paired testes
- 3°C (6°F) lower than core body temperature (temperature necessary for sperm production)
- Temperature is kept constant by two sets of muscles
  - Smooth muscle that wrinkles scrotal skin (**dartos muscle**)
  - Bands of skeletal muscle that elevate the testes (**cremaster muscles**)

Penis
- **Root** and **shaft** end in the **glans penis**
- **Prepuce**, or **foreskin** - the cuff of loose skin covering the glans
  - **Circumcision**: Surgical removal of the foreskin

- **Crura**: The proximal end surrounded by ischiocavernosus muscle; anchors penis to the pubic arch
- **Spongy urethra** and three cylindrical bodies of erectile tissue (spongy network of connective tissue and smooth muscle with vascular spaces)
- **Corpus spongiosum** surrounds the urethra and expands to form the glans and bulb
- **Corpora cavernosa** are paired dorsal erectile bodies
- **Erection**: erectile tissue fills with blood, causing the penis to enlarge and become rigid

Figure 24.1 Male reproductive system, overview

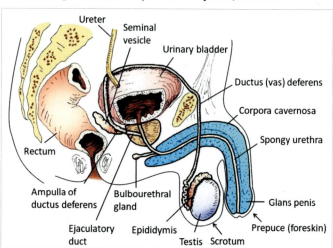

Male Duct System

Epididymis - Nonmotile sperm enter, pass slowly through, and become motile
- **Head**: contains the efferent ductules
- **Duct** of the epididymis
  - Microvilli (stereocilia) absorb testicular fluid and pass nutrients to stored sperm
  - During ejaculation the epididymis contracts, expelling sperm into the ductus deferens

Ductus (Vas) Deferens and Ejaculatory Duct
- **Ductus deferens** passes through the **inguinal canal**
- Expands to form the **ampulla** and then joins the duct of the seminal vesicle to form the **ejaculatory duct**
- Propels sperm from the epididymis to the urethra
- **Vasectomy**: cutting and ligating the ductus deferens, which is a nearly 100% effective form of birth control

Urethra
- Conveys both urine and semen (at different times)
- Has three regions
  - **Prostatic urethra**
  - **Membranous urethra**
  - **Spongy (penile) urethra**

Accessory Glands

Seminal Vesicles
- Produce **viscous alkaline seminal fluid**; 70% of the volume of semen
  - Fructose, ascorbic acid, coagulating enzyme (vesiculase), and prostaglandins
- **Duct of seminal vesicle** joins the ductus deferens to form the **ejaculatory duct**

Prostate
- Encircles part of the urethra inferior to the bladder
- Secretes **milky, slightly acid fluid**:
  - Contains citrate, enzymes, and prostate-specific antigen (PSA)
  - Plays a role in the activation of sperm
  - Enters the prostatic urethra during ejaculation

Bulbourethral Glands (Cowper's Glands)
- Pea-sized glands inferior to the prostate
- Prior to ejaculation, produce **thick, clear mucus**
  - Lubricates the glans penis
  - Neutralizes traces of acidic urine in the urethra

Figure 24.2 Penis, prostate and bladder

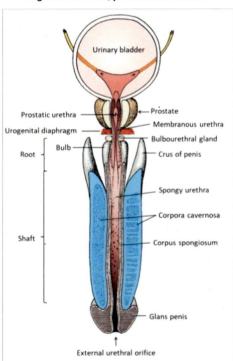

Spermatogenesis
- Sequence of events that produces sperm in the seminiferous tubules of the testes
- Spermatic cells give rise to sperm

- **Mitosis**: Spermatogonia form spermatocytes (are diploid (2*n*); contain 2 sets of chromosomes = 46 chromosomes)
- **Meiosis**: Spermatocytes form spermatids (haploid (*n*); contain 23 chromosomes)
- **Spermiogenesis**: Spermatids become sperm
- Begins at puberty; continues throughout life

Sperm
- **Head**: genetic region; nucleus and helmetlike **acrosome** containing hydrolytic enzymes that enable the sperm to penetrate an egg
- **Midpiece**: metabolic region; mitochondria
- **Tail**: locomotor region; flagellum

Sustentacular (Sertoli) Cells
- Large supporting cells extend through the wall of the tubule and surround developing cells
- Provide nutrients and signals to dividing cells
- Dispose of excess cytoplasm sloughed off during spermiogenesis
- Secrete testicular fluid into lumen for transport of sperm
- Tight junctions form a **blood-testis barrier**

Semen
- **Mixture of sperm and accessory gland secretions**
  - Only 2–5 ml of semen are ejaculated, containing 20–150 million sperm/ml
- Contains nutrients (fructose), protects and activates sperm, and facilitates their movement (e.g., relaxin)
- Prostaglandins in semen
  - Decrease the viscosity of mucus in the cervix
  - Stimulate reverse peristalsis in the uterus
- Alkalinity neutralizes the acid in the male urethra and female vagina
- Antibiotic chemicals destroy certain bacteria
- Clotting factors coagulate semen just after ejaculation, then fibrinolysin liquefies it

Hormonal Regulation of Male Reproductive Function

Hormonal Regulation of Male Reproductive Function
- **Hypothalamic-pituitary-gonadal (HPG) axis**
  - **Hypothalamus** releases **gonadotropin-releasing hormone** (GnRH)
  - GnRH stimulates the **anterior pituitary** to secrete **FSH and LH**
  - FSH causes **sustentacular cells** to release **androgen-binding protein** (ABP), which makes spermatogenic cell receptive to testosterone
  - LH stimulates **interstitial cells** to release **testosterone**
  - Testosterone is the final trigger for spermatogenesis
  - **Feedback inhibition** on the hypothalamus and pituitary results from
    - Rising **levels of testosterone**
    - **Inhibin** (released when sperm count is high)

Testosterone

- Synthesized from cholesterol
- Transformed to exert its effects on some target cells

- **Dihydrotestosterone** (DHT) in the prostate
- **Estrogen** in some neurons in the brain
- Prompts spermatogenesis
- Targets all accessory organs; deficiency leads to atrophy
- Has multiple anabolic effects throughout the body
- Is the basis of the sex drive (libido) in males
- Induces development of **secondary male sex characteristics**
  - Appearance of pubic, axillary, and facial hair
  - Enhanced growth of the chest and deepening of the voice
  - Skin thickens and becomes oily
  - Bones grow and increase in density
  - Skeletal muscles increase in size and mass

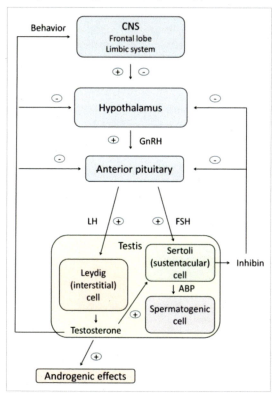

Figure 24.3 Hypothalamus-pituitary-testis axis

Male Sexual Response

- **Erection:** Enlargement and stiffening of the penis from engorgement of erectile tissue with blood
  - Initiated by sexual stimuli, including:
    - Touch and mechanical stimulation of the penis
    - Erotic sights, sounds, and smells

- Can be induced or inhibited by emotions or higher mental activity
- Parasympathetic reflex promotes release of nitric oxide (NO) → causes erectile tissue to fill with blood → expansion of the corpora cavernosa → compresses drainage veins and maintains engorgement
- Corpus spongiosum keeps the urethra open
- **Erectile dysfunction**: inability to attain and/or maintain erection
- **Ejaculation**: Propulsion of semen from the male duct system
  - Sympathetic spinal reflex causes
  - Ducts and accessory glands to contract and empty their contents
  - Bladder sphincter muscle to constrict, preventing the expulsion of urine
  - Bulbospongiosus muscles to undergo a rapid series of contractions

Female Reproductive System

Ovaries
- Produce female gametes (ova)
- Secrete female sex hormones (estrogen and progesterone)
- Held in place by **ovarian**, **suspensory** and **broad ligament** and **mesovarium**
- **Blood supply**: **ovarian arteries** and the ovarian branch of the uterine artery
- Surrounded by a fibrous **tunica albuginea**
  - **Cortex**: ovarian follicles
  - **Medulla**: large blood vessels and nerves
- **Follicle** - Immature egg (**oocyte**) surrounded by
  - **Follicle cells** (one cell layer thick)
  - **Granulosa cells** (when more than one layer is present)
- **Primordial follicle**: follicle cells + oocyte → **Primary follicle**: follicle cells + oocyte → **Secondary follicle**: two or more layers of granulosa cells + oocyte → **Late secondary follicle**: contains fluid-filled space between granulosa cells; coalesces to form a central antrum → **Vesicular (Graafian) follicle**: Fluid-filled antrum forms; follicle bulges from ovary surface
- **Ovulation** - **Ejection of the oocyte** from the ripening follicle
- **Corpus luteum** develops from ruptured follicle after ovulation

Figure 24.4 Ovary, cross-section

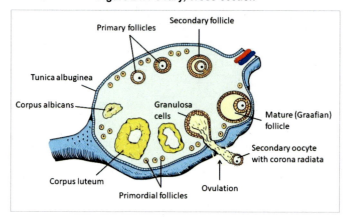

A&P Essentials 4th ed.

Female Duct System

Uterine Tubes
- **Ampulla**: Distal expansion with **infundibulum** near ovary; **usual site of fertilization**
- **Ciliated fimbriae** of infundibulum create currents to move oocyte into uterine tube
- **Isthmus**: constricted region where tube joins uterus
- Oocyte is carried along by peristalsis and ciliary action
- **Nonciliated cells** nourish the oocyte and the sperm

Uterus
- **Body**: major portion
- **Fundus**: rounded superior region
- **Isthmus**: narrowed inferior region
- **Cervix**: narrow neck, or outlet; projects into the vagina
  - **Cervical cana** communicates with vagina via **external os** and uterine cavity via **internal os**
  - **Cervical glands** secrete mucus that blocks sperm entry except during midcycle
- Held in place by **mesometrium, lateral cervical (cardinal), uterosacral and round ligaments**
- **Peritoneal Pouches** - Sacs of peritoneum exist around the uterus
  - **Vesicouterine pouch** is between bladder and uterus
  - **Rectouterine pouch** is between rectum and uterus
- **Uterine Wall** - Three layers
  - **Perimetrium**: serous layer (visceral peritoneum)
  - **Myometrium**: interlacing layers of smooth muscle
  - **Endometrium**: mucosal lining
    - **Stratum functionalis** (functional layer): Changes in response to ovarian hormone cycles; shed during menstruation
    - **Stratum basalis** (basal layer): Forms new functionalis after menstruation; unresponsive to ovarian hormones
- **Blood Supply**
  - **Uterine arteries**: arise from internal iliacs
  - **Arcuate arteries**: in the myometrium
  - **Radial branches** in the endometrium branch into
    - **Spiral arteries** → stratum functionalis
    - **Straight arteries** → stratum basalis
- Spasms of spiral arteries leads to shedding of stratum functionalis

Vagina - Birth canal and organ of copulation
- Extends between the bladder and the rectum from the cervix to the exterior
- Urethra embedded in the anterior wall
- Mucosa near the vaginal orifice forms an incomplete partition called the **hymen**
- **Vaginal fornix**: upper end of the vagina surrounding the cervix

External Genitalia

- a.k.a. vulva or pudendum
- **Mons pubis**: fatty area overlying pubic symphysis

- **Labia majora**: hair-covered, fatty skin folds
- **Labia minora**: skin folds lying within labia majora
- **Vestibule**: recess between labia minora
- **Greater vestibular (Bartholin) glands:** Homologous to the bulbourethral glands; release mucus into the vestibule for lubrication
- **Clitoris:** Erectile tissue hooded by a **prepuce**
  - **Glans clitoris**: exposed portion
- **Perineum:** Diamond-shaped region between the pubic arch and coccyx; bordered by the ischial tuberosities laterally

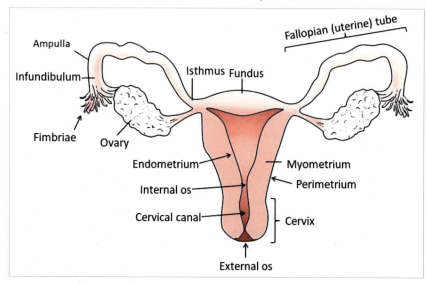

Figure 24.5 Female reproductive system, overview

Mammary (Breast) Glands

- Modified sweat glands consisting of 15–25 **lobes**
- **Areola**: pigmented skin surrounding the nipple
- **Suspensory ligaments**: attach the breast to underlying muscle
- **Lobules** within lobes contain glandular alveoli that produce milk
- Milk → lactiferous ducts → lactiferous sinuses → open to the outside at the nipple

Oogenesis

- Production of female gametes begins in the fetal period
  - **Oogonia** ($2n$ ovarian stem cells) multiply by mitosis and store nutrients
  - **Primary oocytes** develop in primordial follicles; begin meiosis but stall in prophase I
- Each month after puberty, a few primary oocytes are activated → one is selected to resume meiosis I → secondary oocyte
- The **secondary oocyte** arrests in metaphase II and is ovulated
- If penetrated by sperm the second oocyte completes meiosis II, yielding **ovum** (the functional gamete)

A&P Essentials 4th ed.

Female Sex Hormones

Estrogens
- Promote oogenesis and follicle growth in the ovary
- Exert anabolic effects on the female reproductive tract
- Support the rapid but short-lived growth spurt at puberty
- Induce secondary sex characteristics: Growth of the breasts; increased deposit of subcutaneous fat (hips and breasts); widening and lightening of the pelvis
- **Metabolic effects**
  - Maintain low total blood cholesterol and high HDL levels
  - Facilitates calcium uptake

Progesterone
- Works with estrogen to establish and regulate the uterine cycle
- Effects of placental progesterone during pregnancy
- Inhibits uterine motility
- Helps prepare the breasts for lactation

Figure 24.6 Hypothalamus-pituitary-ovary axis

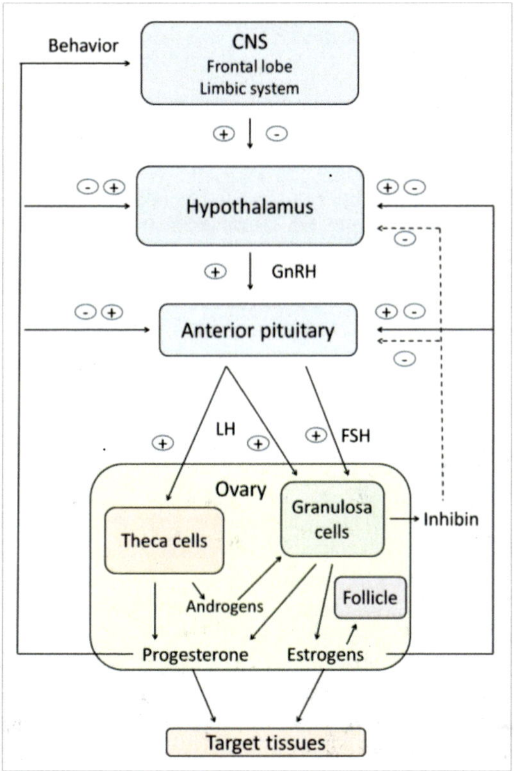

Ovarian Cycle

- Monthly series of events associated with the maturation of an egg
- Two consecutive phases (in a 28-day cycle)

- **Follicular phase**: period of follicle growth (days 1–14)
- **Ovulation** occurs midcycle
- **Luteal phase**: period of corpus luteum activity (days 14–28)

Follicular Phase	**Oogenesis**
	• **Primordial follicle** is activated; enlarges to become a **primary follicle** → **secondary follicle** → **late secondary follicle** → **vesicular follicle** - follicle bulges from the external surface of the ovary
	• The primary oocyte completes meiosis I
	Hormonal interactions
	• GnRH → release of FSH and LH
	• FSH and LH → growth of several follicles, and estrogen release
	• ↑ estrogen levels
	  • Inhibit the release of FSH and LH
	  • Stimulate synthesis and storage of FSH and LH
	  • Enhance further estrogen output
	• Estrogen output by the vesicular follicle increases
	• High estrogen levels have a positive feedback effect on the pituitary at midcycle

Ovulation	**Oogenesis**
	• Ovary wall ruptures and expels the secondary oocyte with its corona radiata
	• **Mittelschmerz**: twinge of pain sometimes felt at ovulation
	• 1–2% of ovulations release more than one secondary oocyte, which, if fertilized, results in fraternal twins
	Hormonal interactions
	• Sudden **LH surge** at day 14
	• Effects of LH surge
	  • Completion of meiosis I (secondary oocyte continues on to metaphase II)
	  • Triggers ovulation
	  • Transforms ruptured follicle into corpus luteum

Luteal phase	**Oogenesis** • Ruptured follicle collapses; granulosa cells and internal thecal cells form corpus luteum • **Corpus luteum** secretes progesterone and estrogen • If **no pregnancy**, the corpus luteum degenerates into a corpus albicans in 10 days • If **pregnancy** occurs, corpus luteum produces hormones until the placenta takes over at about 3 months **Hormonal interactions** • Corpus luteum produces **inhibin**, **progesterone**, and **estrogen** • These hormones inhibit FSH and LH release • Declining LH and FSH ends luteal activity and inhibits follicle development

- **Days 26–28**: corpus luteum degenerates and ovarian hormone levels drop sharply → ends the blockade of FSH and LH → cycle starts anew

Establishing the Ovarian Cycle
- During childhood, **until puberty**
  - Ovaries secrete small amounts of estrogens
  - Estrogen inhibits release of GnRH
- **At puberty**
  - Leptin from adipose tissue decreases the estrogen inhibition
  - GnRH, FSH, and LH are released
- In about four years, an adult cyclic pattern is achieved and **menarche** occurs

Uterine (Menstrual) Cycle

- Cyclic changes in endometrium in response to ovarian hormones
  - Days 1–5: **menstrual phase**
  - Days 6–14: **proliferative** (preovulatory) **phase**
  - Days 15–28: **secretory** (postovulatory) **phase** (constant 14-day length)

Menstrual phase	**Hormone levels** • Ovarian hormones are at their lowest levels • Gonadotropins are beginning to rise **Effect on uterus** • Stratum functionalis is shed and the menstrual flow occurs
Proliferative phase	**Hormone levels** • Estrogen levels prompt generation of new functional layer and increased synthesis of progesterone receptors in endometrium **Effect on uterus** • Glands enlarge and spiral arteries increase in number

Secretory phase	**Hormone levels**
	• Progesterone levels prompt further development of endometrium
	• If fertilization does not occur
	  • Corpus luteum degenerates
	  • Progesterone levels fall
	Effect on uterus
	• Glandular secretion of glycogen
	• Formation of the cervical mucus plug
	• If fertilization does not occur
	  • Spiral arteries kink and spasm Endometrial cells begin to die
	  • Spiral arteries constrict again, then relax and open wide
	  • Rush of blood fragments weakened capillary beds and the functional layer sloughs

Female Sex Response

- Initiated by touch and psychological stimuli
- The clitoris, vaginal mucosa, and breasts engorge with blood

- Vestibular gland secretions lubricate the vestibule
- Orgasm is accompanied by muscle tension, increase in pulse rate and blood pressure, and rhythmic contractions of the uterus
- Females do not have a refractory period after orgasm and can experience multiple orgasms in a single sexual experience
- Orgasm is not essential for conception

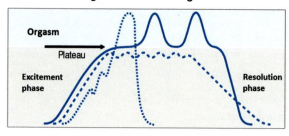

Figure 24.7 Female orgasm

Pregnancy

Pregnancy: Events that occur from fertilization until the infant is born
- **Conceptus**: the developing offspring
- **Gestation period**: time from the last menstrual period until birth (~280 days)
- **Embryo**: conceptus from fertilization through week 8
- **Fetus**: conceptus from week 9 through birth

Under **clinical aspects**, pregnancy is divided into three **trimesters of unequal length**:
1. The **first trimester extends from conception until the end of week 12**. At the end of the first trimester all body organs and systems have been formed, and the placenta is developed enough to keep the baby alive.
2. The **second trimester** extends from the beginning of week 13 until the end of week 28. By the end of the second trimester, more than 90% of babies can survive outside of the uterus if born prematurely.
3. The **third trimester** extends from the beginning of week 29 through week 40 (or delivery).

Fertilization: when the sperm's chromosomes combine with those of a secondary oocyte to form a fertilized egg (zygote)
- Ejaculated **sperm**
  - Leak out of the vagina immediately after deposition
  - Are destroyed by the acidic vaginal environment
  - Fail to make it through the cervix
  - Are dispersed in the uterine cavity or destroyed by phagocytes
  - Few (100 to a few thousand) reach the uterine tubes
- The oocyte is viable for 12 to 24 hours
- Sperm is viable 24 to 48 hours after ejaculation
- For fertilization to occur, coitus must occur no more than
  - Two days before ovulation
  - 24 hours after ovulation

Embryonic Development

- **Cleavage** - Mitotic divisions of **zygote**
- First cleavage at 36 hours → two daughter cells (**blastomeres**)
- At 72 hours → **morula** (16 or more cells)
- At day 3 or 4, the embryo of ~100 cells (**blastocyst**) has reached the uterus
- **Blastocyst**: fluid-filled hollow sphere
  - **Trophoblast cells**
    - Display factors that are immunosuppressive
    - Participate in placenta formation
  - **Inner cell mass**
    - Becomes the embryonic disc (→ embryo and three of the embryonic membranes)
- **Implantation**
  - Blastocyst floats for 2–3 days
  - Implantation begins 6–7 days after ovulation
  - Trophoblast adheres to a site with the proper receptors and chemical signals
  - Inflammatory-like response occurs in the endometrium
  - Trophoblasts proliferate and form two distinct layers
    - **Cytotrophoblast** (cellular trophoblast): inner layer of cells
    - **Syncytiotrophoblast**: cells in the outer layer lose their plasma membranes, invade and digest the endometrium
  - The implanted blastocyst is covered over by endometrial cells
  - Implantation is completed by the twelfth day after ovulation

The embryo has **three germ layers** from which all tissues and organs derive:
1. The outer **ectoderm** (*ecto-* outside, *-derm* skin) forms the nervous system and the epidermis of the skin
2. The inner **endoderm** (*endo-* inside, *-derm* skin) forms the epithelial linings of the digestive, respiratory, and urogenital systems, and their associated glands
3. The middle **mesoderm** (*meso-* middle, *-derm* skin) forms all other tissues, such as muscles and internal organs

Embryonic membranes
- The **chorion** is the outermost of the **embryonic membranes**. It helps to form the placenta and encloses the embryonic body and all other membranes
- The **amnion** forms the transparent sac containing the embryo. It is filled with **amniotic fluid** that provides a buoyant environment, which protects the embryo from physical trauma
- The **yolk sac** forms part of the gut of the embryo and produces the earliest blood cells and blood vessels. It is also the origin of germ cells that migrate into the embryo to seed the **gonads** (testicles and ovaries)
- The **allantois** forms the base for the **umbilical cord**. It also becomes part of the urinary bladder of the baby

Placenta (also known as **afterbirth**)
- Connects the developing fetus to the uterus and creates an interface for the exchange of nutrients, gases (oxygen, carbon dioxide), and waste products between the blood of the fetus and the mother
- Produces hormones that keep the fetus alive and stop the ovaries from producing new eggs while still pregnant
- Has a fetal part (**chorion**) and a maternal part (**decidua**)

- The **umbilical cord** contains blood vessels that transport blood from the fetus to the placenta (**umbilical arteries**) or from the placenta to the fetus (**umbilical vein**)

Pregnancy Hormones

Human chorionic gonadotropin (hCG)
- Secreted by trophoblast cells, later the chorion
- Prompts corpus luteum to continue secretion of progesterone and estrogen
- hCG levels rise until the end of the second month, then decline as the placenta begins to secrete progesterone and estrogen
- **Estrogens** and **progesterone** are vital for the development of the uterus and the fetus.
- **Inhibin** stops the anterior pituitary from releasing FSH to make sure no additional follicle can develop during the pregnancy
- **Relaxin** causes pelvic ligaments and the pubic symphysis to soften and relax
- **Human placenta lactogen** (hPL) supports estrogens and progesterone in getting the breast gland ready for lactation. It also promotes fetal growth and causes the maternal metabolism to burn fatty acids in tissues other than nervous tissue. This so-called glucose-sparing effect saves glucose for the nervous system of the mother and the baby
- **Human chorionic thyrotropin** (hCT) increases the metabolic rate of the mother. Due to the heat created by the increased metabolic activity of the cells, pregnant women often feel warm and sweat more even when the environment is cold

Delivery

Delivery or **parturition** is the process of giving birth. Most births happen within 15 days of the expected **due date**, which is **280 days from the first day of the last period before pregnancy**.

There are **three stages of labor**:
1. The **dilation stage** extends from the onset of labor to the time when the cervix is fully dilated (about 10 cm; 4 inches) by the baby's head.
2. The **expulsion stage** extends from full dilation until the time the infant is delivered. **Crowning** occurs when the baby's head distends the vulva. When the baby is in the **vertex** or **head-first position**, the skull acts as a wedge to dilate the cervix, vagina, and vulva. Once the head has been delivered, the rest of the baby follows much more easily. After birth, the umbilical cord is clamped and cut.
3. During the **placental stage**, uterine contractions cause detachment of the placenta from the uterine wall. This allows for delivery of the placenta and the membranes (afterbirth).

- The **average full-term baby weighs about 7.5 pounds**
- The **average length** of full-term babies is **20 inches** (18–22 inches)

Lactation is the production of milk by the mammary glands
- Milk production is stimulated by the **prolactin** from the anterior pituitary
- Oxytocin causes the so-called **letdown reflex** resulting in the release of milk from the glands of both breasts

Genetic Sex

- **Women** have **two sex chromosomes** (**XX**) in each body cell; their gametes (**oocytes**) have **one X chromosomes** each
- **Men** have **one X chromosome and one Y chromosome** in each body cell; sperm

cells contain either one X chromosome or one Y chromosome
- **The genetic sex of the offspring is determined by the sex chromosome carried by the sperm**
  - If an egg is fertilized by an X sperm, the zygote has two X chromosomes and the baby is genetically female.
  - If an egg is fertilized by a Y sperm, the zygote has one X chromosome and one Y chromosome and the baby is genetically male.

Table 24.1 Terms Associated with Pregnancy and Birth

Term	Meaning	Example(s)
gravida	pregnant woman	*nulligravida* = a woman who has never been pregnant
		primigravida = a woman who is pregnant for the first time or has been pregnant once before
		multigravida = a women who is pregnant for the second time or has been pregnant at least twice
para	a woman who has given birth at least once	*nullipara* = a woman who has never born a child
		primipara = a woman who has given birth once
		multipara = a woman who has given birth twice or more
parous	having given birth one or more times	*nulliparous* or *nonparous* = never having borne a child
		primiparous = giving or having given birth for the first time
		multiparous = having given birth more than once
natal	relating to birth (from the baby's point of view)	*prenatal* or *antenatal* = (occurring) before birth
		postnatal = (occurring) after birth
		perinatal = relating to the period from about five months (week 20) before birth to one month after birth
		neonatal = relating to the first four week (28 days) after birth
antepartum, prepartum	occurring before delivery (from the mother's point of view)	*antepartum bleeding* = bleeding after the 24th week of gestation but before delivery
peripartum	occurring during the last month of pregnancy and the first five months after	*peripartum cardiomyopathy* = uncommon form of heart failure that occurs during the last month of preg-

	delivery (from the mother's point of view)	nancy or up to five months after delivery
postpartum, puerperal	occurring after delivery (from the mother's point of view)	*postpartum period* or *puerperium* = the first six weeks after delivery

Birth control

Birth control or **contraception** is a term for methods used to prevent pregnancy.

- **Hormonal birth control** includes then use of birth control pills, hormone injections or skin patches, hormone implants under the skin, and vaginal rings. Some IUDs (see below) also release small amounts of hormone.
- **Intrauterine devices (IUDs)** are inserted into the uterine cavity. The prevent implantation of a fertilized egg by causing a local inflammation (copper IUD) or the release of levonorgestrel (hormone IUD).
- **Barrier methods** are physical contraceptives that prevent the sperm from getting into the uterus. They include condoms, diaphragms, sponges, and cervical caps.
- **Emergency contraceptives** (so-called Plan B or **morning-after pill**) are used to prevent pregnancy after unprotected sex or failure of barrier methods, e.g., condom rupture. The pill contains 1.5 mg levonorgestrel.
- **Permanent birth control** or **sterilization** can be used by women (**tubal ligation**) or men (**vasectomy**).